# Pediatric Cancer Genetics

# Pediatric Cancer Genetics

NATHANIEL H. ROBIN, MD
Director of the Genetics Residency Programs
The University of Alabama at Birmingham
Birmingham, Alabama

MEAGAN B. FARMER, MS, CGC
Director of the Cancer Genetic Counseling Program
Departments of Genetics
The University of Alabama at Birmingham
Birmingham, Alabama

ELSEVIER

# ELSEVIER

3251 Riverport Lane
St. Louis, Missouri 63043

*Content Strategist:* Kayla Wolfe
*Content Development Manager:* Taylor Ball
*Content Development Specialist:* Casey Potter
*Publishing Services Manager:* Deepthi Unni
*Project Manager:* Janish Ashwin Paul
*Designer:* Renee Deunow

Printed in United States of America

Last digit is the print number:　9　8　7　6　5　4　3　2　1

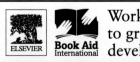

# List of Contributors

**Elizabeth Alva, MD, MSPH**
Director, Pediatric Cancer Predisposition Screening
    Clinic
Pediatric Hematology and Oncology
The University of Alabama at Birmingham
Birmingham, Alabama

**J. Austin Hamm, MD**
Medical Director of Pediatric Genetics
East Tennessee Children's Hospital
Children's Hospital Genetics Center
Knoxville, Tennessee

**Joseph H. Chewning, MD**
Clinical Director, Lowder Pediatric Blood and Marrow
    Transplant Program
The University of Alabama at Birmingham
Birmingham, Alabama

**Alexandra Cutillo, MA**
The University of Alabama at Birmingham
Birmingham, Alabama

**Katie Farmer, MS, CGC**
Clinical Genetics Center
Tallahassee Memorial Hospital
Tallahassee, Florida

**Meagan B. Farmer, MS, CGC**
Director of the Cancer Genetic Counseling Program
Departments of Genetics and Pediatrics
The University of Alabama at Birmingham
Birmingham, Alabama

**Alicia Gomes, MS,CGC**
UAB Medical Genomics Laboratory
Department of Genetics
The University of Alabama at Birmingham
Birmingham, Alabama

**Sonja Higgins, MS, CGC**
Murrells Inlet, South Carolina

**Anna C.E. Hurst, MD, MS**
Assistant Professor, Department of Genetics
The University of Alabama at Birmingham
Birmingham, Alabama

**Michael G. Hurst, MD**
Assistant Professor
UAB Center for Palliative and Supportive Care
The University of Alabama at Birmingham
Birmingham, Alabama

**Avi Madan-Swain, PhD**
Professor of Pediatrics
Director, Hope and Cope Psychosocial and Education
    Program
UAB Division of Pediatric Hematology-Oncology
The University of Alabama at Birmingham
Birmingham, Alabama

**Nathaniel H. Robin, MD**
Director of the Genetics Residency Programs
The University of Alabama at Birmingham
Birmingham, Alabama

**Theresa V. Strong, PhD**
Adjunct Professor
Department of Genetics
University of Alabama at Birmingham
Birmingham, Alabama

**Kimberly Whelan, MD, MSPH**
Associate Professor
Division of Pediatric Hematology-Oncology
Department of Pediatrics
The University of Alabama at Birmingham
Birmingham, Alabama

**Bruce R. Korf, MD, PhD**
Wayne H. and Sara Crews Finley Chair in Medical
    Genetics
Professor and Chair, Department of Genetics
The University of Alabama at Birmingham
Birmingham, Alabama

# Preface

The past decade has seen genetic discovery proceeding at a staggering rate. This has included dramatic advances in understanding the underlying pathobiology of disease, as well as greatly enhanced the ability to detect genetic alterations through increased capabilities in genetic testing technologies. Although these advances have impacted nearly every area of medicine, nowhere has it been more prominent than the field of cancer genetics. An ever-growing number of genes have been implicated in hereditary cancer susceptibility, and scientists and clinicians are working diligently to elucidate the implications for patients. Patients or their parents want to know why cancer occurred in the first place, whether it might occur again, and who else in the family might be at risk. Genetic evaluation and potentially genetic testing may be able to address these questions. However, patients are best served when genetic evaluation occurs by genetics professionals who work as part of a multidisciplinary team.

Although cancer genetic counseling by a genetics professional is available in most academic cancer centers, such services are less commonly available in pediatric oncology. Most cases of pediatric cancer occur sporadically, with no significant findings in the medical history, family history, or physical examination to suggest an underlying hereditary cancer syndrome. However, it is estimated that ~10% of pediatric cancer cases do, in fact, have an underlying hereditary cause. Furthermore, in a review of patients/families followed in a pediatric cancer survivors' clinic, almost a third (29%) had findings that warranted a genetics evaluation.[1] The same study found that before the introduction of genetic services, only 6% of these patients/families were evaluated by genetics. Although this is only one study at one center, these results are likely similar for most pediatric oncology centers.

Pediatricians are typically very knowledgeable about medical genetics in the context of genetic syndromes and inborn errors of metabolism. However, in our experience, they seem to be less familiar in the context of cancer genetics. Why is this? Cancer genetics is a relatively new field and was not part of the training for most pediatric oncologists. The priority of genetic evaluation and testing may also seem low to clinicians because they are entirely focused on treating a child's cancer. Unfortunately, this is to the detriment of patients and their families. The results of a genetic evaluation may significantly affect how the cancer is treated, assist in planning future surveillance of the patient, and have implications for at-risk family members.

The goal of this book is to provide a resource on cancer genetics for pediatric oncologists and all providers who care for children with cancer. This is a comprehensive overview of the many facets of pediatric cancer genetics. In the following chapters we will review the epidemiology and biology of cancer, describe the genetic evaluation process and role of genetic counselors, highlight examples of syndromes that present in childhood and increase susceptibility to cancer, discuss the genetic evaluation process in context of the multidisciplinary care of children with cancer, consider the ethical and legal issues of genetic testing in children, and provide illustrative case examples. It is not an in-depth review of any single topic—by reading this book, we do not expect anyone to become a cancer geneticist or genetic counselor. We intend to cover each topic in a manner that is accessible for all clinicians and provides a basic level of knowledge.

In summary, thousands of children and adolescents are diagnosed with cancer each year, and many of these individuals could benefit from genetics evaluations. It is unrealistic to expect referring pediatricians and/or oncology teams to conduct thorough genetics evaluations, coordinate and interpret testing that is increasingly complex in nature, and make medical recommendations for patients and their families. However, it is not only appropriate but also manageable for pediatricians and oncology teams to be aware of the medical/family history clues that may suggest genetics evaluation is appropriate, understand and be able to explain to families why genetics evaluation may be beneficial, and make a referral to a genetics team. This book aims to allow providers who care for children with cancer to feel proficient in this role.

**Nathaniel H. Robin, MD**
**Meagan B. Farmer, MS, CGC**

## REFERENCES

1. Knapke S, Nagarajan R, Correll J, Kent D, Burns K. Hereditary cancer risk assessment in a pediatric oncology follow-up clinic. *Pediatr Blood Cancer*. 2011;58:85–89.

## FURTHER READING

1. American Cancer Society. *Cancer Facts & Figures 2015*. Atlanta: American Cancer Society; 2015.
2. National Cancer Institute. *Cancer Genetics Risk Assessment and Counseling-for Health Professionals*. NIH; 2015.

3. Knapke S, Zelley K, Nichols K, Kohlmann W, Schiffman J. Identification, management, and evaluation of children with cancer-predisposition syndromes. In: *Pediatric Oncology Educational Book*. 2012.
4. Hamm J, Mikhail F, Hollenbeck D, Farmer M, Robin N. Incidental detection of cancer predisposition gene copy number variations by array comparative genomic hybridization. *J Pediatr*. (n.d.).

# Contents

# CHAPTER 1

# Epidemiology of Childhood Cancer

KIMBERLY WHELAN, MD, MSPH • ELIZABETH ALVA, MD, MSPH

## INTRODUCTION

Approximately 16,400 children and adolescents are diagnosed with a cancer every year in the United States. While childhood cancer remains relatively rare, it is also the leading cause of disease-related deaths in children and adolescents.[1] There are many differences between adult and childhood malignancies, including incidence, risk factors, and prognosis. One of the most important differences is the basis of classification of cancer types. Most adult cancers are categorized based on their site of origin. In pediatric oncology, cancers are classified based on their histology.[2]

Data about the epidemiology of childhood cancer come from multiple sources. Because of the incomplete nature of cancer registries among the states, the exact number of incident cases of pediatric cancer each year is unknown. One of the most comprehensive databases for cancer incidence is the Surveillance, Epidemiology and End Results (SEER) program of the National Cancer Institute. The SEER program reports high-quality, long-term, population-based incidence data covering ~28% of the population of the United States. Data on incidence trends in the SEER database extend back to 1975 and can allow for the examination of the pediatric cancer incidence trends over time. The North American Association of Central Cancer Registries (NAACCR) is the more recently established registry, which reports incidence data from 1995 onward. In the NAACCR the cancer registries that participate in the SEER program, as well as the registries that participate in the Centers for Disease Control and Prevention's Nation Program of Cancer Registries, are included. The NAACR covers up to 95% of the US population. However, both the SEER and NAACCR data reporting of incidence data lag behind the current year because of the time needed for data collection, aggregation, and dissemination. Descriptive epidemiology data reported in this chapter come from both the SEER program and NAACR as well as recent publications from the American Cancer Society.[3–5]

Other important sources of information about childhood cancer include cooperative groups, such as the Children's Oncology Group (COG). The COG has over 220 member institutions, and 90% of all children and adolescents diagnosed with cancer in the United States are treated at a COG institution. In 2001, COG launched the Childhood Cancer Research Network (CCRN). The CCRN was a North American pediatric cancer registry available to patients and families diagnosed at a COG institution in the United States and Canada.[6] More recently, Project:EveryChild was initiated by the COG. This innovative study hopes to store biologic tumor specimens and track patient outcome data; therefore outcomes and biologic features may be more closely linked, even for the most rare tumor types.[1]

Epidemiology is defined as the study of the distribution and determinants of health-related events, in this case childhood cancer, with the hopes of applying the knowledge learned.[7] This chapter aims to explore the descriptive epidemiology of childhood cancer, including incidence, mortality, and survival rates for both childhood and adolescent cancer. This will be followed by a discussion of the possible causes and determining factors related to childhood cancer.

## PEDIATRIC CANCER INCIDENCE BY AGE AND CANCER TYPE

In 2014, it is estimated that there will be 15,780 incident cases of pediatric cancer diagnosed in the United States among children and adolescents aged 0–19 years, with 10,450 cases in children aged 0–14 years and 5330 cases in adolescents aged 15–19 years.[5] Altogether, these cases represent only 1% of all new cancers diagnosed in the United States. In the United States, 1 of approximately every 408 children will be diagnosed with cancer before the age of 15 years and 1 of approximately every 285 children will be diagnosed with cancer before the age of 20 years.[5] The most common cancer types vary by age group and are detailed in Figs. 1.1 and 1.2. In the 0–14 years age group, acute lymphocytic leukemia (ALL) makes up the majority of cases with an estimated 2670 cases (26%), followed by brain and central nervous system (CNS) tumors with 2240 cases

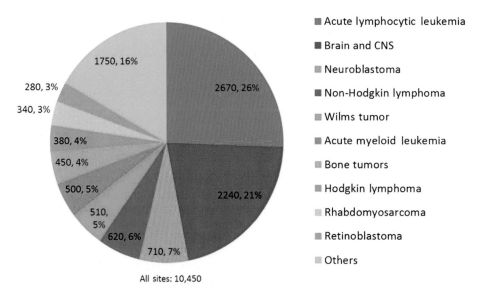

FIG. 1.1 Estimated incident cases of childhood cancers for 2014 in the United States, ages 0–14 years. Estimates are for malignant cancers only and are rounded to the nearest 10. (Data from Ward E, Desantis C, Robbins A, Kohler B, Jemal A. Childhood and adolescent cancer statistics, 2014. *CA Cancer J Clin*. 2014;64:83–103.)

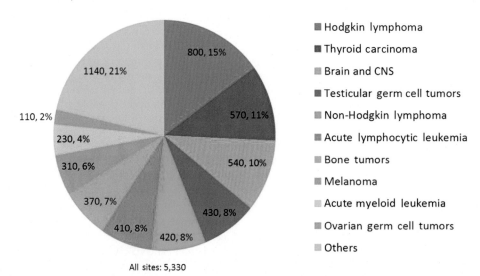

FIG. 1.2 Estimated incident cases of childhood cancers for 2014 in the United States, ages 15–19 years. Estimates are for malignant cancers only and are rounded to the nearest 10. (Data from Ward E, Desantis C, Robbins A, Kohler B, Jemal A. Childhood and adolescent cancer statistics, 2014. *CA Cancer J Clin*. 2014;64:83–103.)

(21%), and neuroblastoma with 710 cases (7%). Non-Hodgkin's lymphoma makes up an additional 620 cases (6%) in the 0–14 years age group, followed closely by Wilm's tumor with 510 cases (5%). In the 15–19 years age group, the most common cancer type is Hodgkin's lymphoma with 800 cases (15%), followed by thyroid carcinoma with 570 cases (11%), and brain and CNS tumors with 540 cases (10%). Testicular germ cell tumors are the fourth most common diagnosis in the 15–19 years age group with 430 cases (8%), followed by non-Hodgkin's lymphoma with 420 cases (8%).

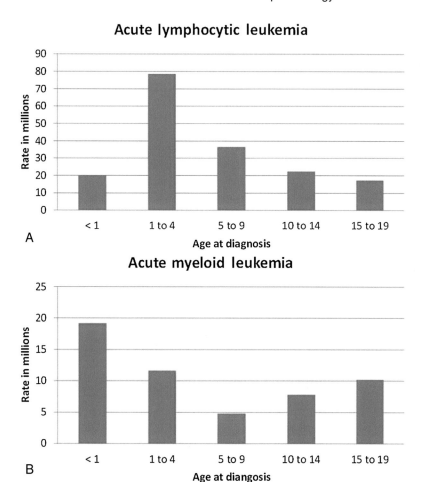

FIG. 1.3 Age-specific incidence rates for acute lymphocytic leukemia **(A)** and acute myeloid leukemia **(B)**, United States, 2009–13. (Data from Ward E, Desantis C, Robbins A, Kohler B, Jemal A. Childhood and adolescent cancer statistics, 2014. *CA Cancer J Clin*. 2014;64:83–103.)

Within each specific type of pediatric cancer, there is also variation in incidence by age. For ALL, there is a peak in incidence in the 1–4 years age group, whereas acute myeloid leukemia demonstrates a more bimodal distribution in incidence, with the highest incidence occurring in the less than 1 year age group and second, smaller, peak in 15–19 years age group (Fig. 1.3). Both Hodgkin's and non-Hodgkin's lymphomas show a steady increase in incidence with age (Fig. 1.4). For embryonal tumors, including Wilm's tumor, retinoblastoma, neuroblastoma, and hepatoblastoma, the incidence is highest in the younger age groups and steadily declines with increasing age (Fig. 1.5). For retinoblastoma and hepatoblastoma, incident cases almost always occur before the age of 5 years, although rare cases can occur at older age groups. In bone tumors, both osteosarcoma and Ewing's

sarcoma, the incidence increases with increasing age (Fig. 1.6). However, for rhabdomyosarcoma, the peak incidence occurs in the 1–4 years age group and then declines with increasing age (Fig. 1.6).

## PEDIATRIC CANCER INCIDENCE BY GENDER

Incidence rates for all pediatric cancers combined are higher in males at ~187 per million compared with females at ~170 per million. There are several cancer types where the incidence rates are dramatically different between males and females. Non-Hodgkin's lymphoma has a significantly higher incidence rate in males (15.2 per million) than in females (7.9 per million). Males also have a higher incidence of malignant

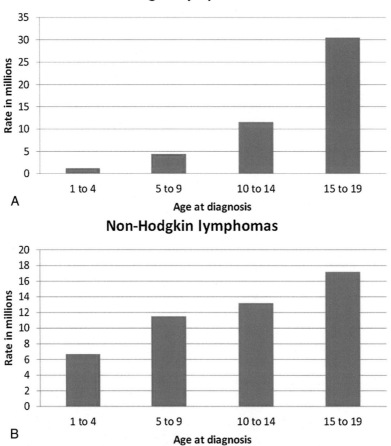

FIG. 1.4 Age-specific incidence rates for Hodgkin's **(A)** and non-Hodgkin's **(B)** lymphomas, United States, 2009–13. (Data from Howlader N, Noone AM, Krapcho M, et al., eds. *SEER Cancer Statistics Review, 1975–2013*. Bethesda, MD: National Cancer Institute; April 2016. http://seer.cancer.gov/csr/1975_2013/, based on November 2015 SEER data submission, posted to the SEER web site.)

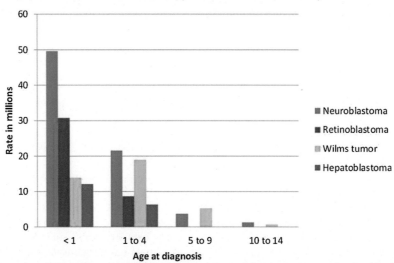

FIG. 1.5 Age-specific incidence rates of embryonal tumors, United States, 2009–13. (Data from Howlader N, Noone AM, Krapcho M, et al., eds. *SEER Cancer Statistics Review, 1975–2013*. Bethesda, MD: National Cancer Institute; April 2016. http://seer.cancer.gov/csr/1975_2013/, based on November 2015 SEER data submission, posted to the SEER web site.)

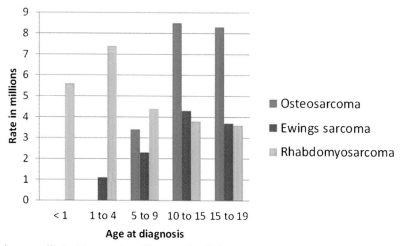

FIG. 1.6 Age-specific incidence rates of bone and soft tissue sarcomas, United States, 2009–13. (Data from Howlader N, Noone AM, Krapcho M, et al., eds. *SEER Cancer Statistics Review, 1975–2013*. Bethesda, MD: National Cancer Institute; April 2016. http://seer.cancer.gov/csr/1975_2013/, based on November 2015 SEER data submission, posted to the SEER web site.)

gonadal tumors than females with an incidence rate of 10 per million for testicular germ cell tumors versus an incidence rate of 4.5 per million for ovarian germ cell tumors. However, the incidence rates for thyroid carcinoma are dramatically higher in females with a rate of 14.5 per million in females compared with 3.2 per million in males. These differences in the incidence rates can be seen among males and females of all races/ethnicities, with the exception of malignant gonadal tumors, which show a higher incidence in black females compared with black males. Detailed incidence rates for the major International Classification of Childhood Cancer (ICCC) subtypes by gender and race/ethnicity can be found in Table 1.1.

## PEDIATRIC CANCER INCIDENCE BY RACE/ETHNICITY

Pediatric cancer incidence is highest in the non-Hispanic white population, followed closely by the Hispanic population (Table 1.1). Incidence rates for non-Hispanic blacks and Asian/Pacific Islanders are similar and notably lower than both the non-Hispanic white and Hispanic populations. American Indians and Alaska Natives have the lowest incidence of pediatric cancer of all the races/ethnicities. Among the different cancer types, there are some striking differences in incidences among the racial/ethnic groups. For Ewing's sarcoma, the incidence rate is substantially lower in the non-Hispanic black population, both males and

females, compared with all other populations. The incidence of testicular germ cell tumors is also much lower in non-Hispanic black males than in all other racial/ethnic groups. In addition, pediatric melanoma cases are significantly higher in the non-Hispanic white population than in any other ethnic group. The etiology behind the difference in cancer incidence among ethnicities has not been elucidated thus far. Further details on incidence rates for the major ICCC subtypes by gender and racial/ethnic groups can be found in Table 1.1.

## TRENDS IN PEDIATRIC CANCER INCIDENCE OVER TIME

Between 1975 and 2013, the incidence rate of all pediatric cancers combined has been increasing at an average rate of 0.6% annually.[3] Among the different types of cancer, increased incidence rates have occurred in ALL, brain and CNS tumors, non-Hodgkin's lymphoma, and soft tissue sarcomas (Fig. 1.7). For brain and CNS tumors, a significant increase in incidence rates was seen between 1983 and 1986 and is thought to be secondary to the introduction of magnetic resonance imaging as well as new surgical biopsy techniques that allowed for better identification of tumors. Subsequent to this significant increase, the incidence rates for brain and CNS tumors have remained fairly steady, with a nonstatistically significant increase in incidence rates of only 0.2% per year. The incidence rates of Hodgkin's lymphomas have actually decreased between 1975 and 2013, with

**TABLE 1.1**
Pediatric Cancer Incidence Rates by Gender and Race/Ethnicity, Ages 0–19 Years, United States, 2008–12

| | ALL RACES | | NON-HISPANIC WHITE | | NON-HISPANIC BLACK | | HISPANIC | | ASIAN/PACIFIC ISLANDER | |
|---|---|---|---|---|---|---|---|---|---|---|
| | Male | Female | Male | Female | Male | Female | Male | Female | Male | Female |
| All ICCC sites | 186.6 | 170.4 | 198.1 | 181.6 | 143.3 | 133.7 | 182.1 | 163.1 | 148.6 | 134.3 |
| Leukemia | 51.9 | 43.6 | 51.1 | 43.2 | 33.8 | 26.6 | 63.4 | 53.3 | 47.2 | 39.0 |
| Acute lymphocytic leukemia | 38.2 | 30.5 | 38.2 | 30.6 | 21.4 | 15.4 | 48.0 | 39.9 | 33.9 | 25.9 |
| Acute myeloid leukemia | 8.0 | 8.0 | 7.6 | 7.8 | 7.0 | 6.8 | 8.9 | 8.5 | 7.8 | 8.6 |
| Lymphomas | 31.3 | 22.4 | 33.7 | 24.2 | 27.0 | 19.2 | 27.0 | 19.7 | 24.1 | 16.8 |
| Hodgkin's lymphoma | 12.7 | 12.0 | 14.0 | 13.7 | 11.1 | 10.3 | 10.8 | 9.4 | 7.5 | 6.5 |
| Non-Hodgkin's lymphoma | 15.2 | 7.9 | 16.2 | 7.8 | 14.8 | 7.9 | 12.0 | 7.4 | 13.7 | 8.1 |
| Brain and CNS | 33.5 | 29.6 | 38.4 | 33.4 | 27.3 | 25.1 | 25.6 | 23.6 | 22.2 | 18.0 |
| Ependymoma | 2.9 | 2.3 | 2.9 | 2.5 | 2.4 | 1.9 | 2.9 | 2.4 | 2.8 | 1.3 |
| Astrocytoma | 16.6 | 15.6 | 19.8 | 18.1 | 13.4 | 12.7 | 11.5 | 11.9 | 9.4 | 8.8 |
| CNS embryonal tumors | 7.3 | 5.0 | 8.3 | 5.4 | 5.2 | 3.8 | 6.4 | 4.6 | 5.5 | 4.1 |
| Other gliomas | 5.5 | 5.7 | 6.3 | 6.6 | 4.9 | 5.1 | 3.8 | 3.9 | 3.9 | 3.5 |
| Neuroblastoma and ganglioneuroblastoma | 8.6 | 7.8 | 10.3 | 9.3 | 7.2 | 7.2 | 5.6 | 4.8 | 6.9 | 5.6 |
| Retinoblastoma | 3.1 | 3.3 | 2.8 | 3.0 | 3.3 | 3.6 | 3.4 | 3.6 | 2.4 | 3.6 |
| Wilm's tumor | 5.8 | 6.9 | 6.3 | 7.4 | 6.8 | 8.2 | 4.4 | 5.3 | 2.4 | 3.8 |
| Hepatic tumors | 2.9 | 2.0 | 2.7 | 1.9 | 2.2 | 1.7 | 3.1 | 2.3 | 3.6 | 1.9 |
| Bone tumors | 9.6 | 7.8 | 10.0 | 8.1 | 7.6 | 6.6 | 10.0 | 7.4 | 7.7 | 7.3 |
| Osteosarcoma | 5.5 | 4.5 | 5.1 | 4.2 | 6.3 | 5.3 | 5.8 | 4.6 | 4.1 | 4.6 |
| Ewing's sarcoma | 3.2 | 2.4 | 4.0 | 3.1 | 0.4 | 0.4 | 3.1 | 2.0 | 2.5 | 2.0 |
| Rhabdomyosarcoma | 5.2 | 4.3 | 5.4 | 4.3 | 5.9 | 4.7 | 4.5 | 3.8 | 3.1 | 3.4 |
| Testicular germ cell tumors | 10.0 | | 10.6 | | 1.1 | | 15.1 | | 5.9 | |
| Ovarian germ cell tumors | | 4.5 | | 3.5 | | 5.1 | | 6.2 | | 4.7 |
| Thyroid carcinoma | 3.2 | 14.5 | 3.7 | 17.0 | 1.5 | 5.1 | 2.4 | 14.1 | 3.2 | 15.1 |
| Melanoma | 3.5 | 5.3 | 5.1 | 7.9 | 0.5 | 0.6 | 1.0 | 1.9 | 0.7 | 1.0 |

CNS, central nervous system; ICCC, International Classification of Childhood Cancers.
Rates are per 1,000,000 and are standardized to the 2000 US standard population.
Data from North American Association of Central Cancer Registries Inc.

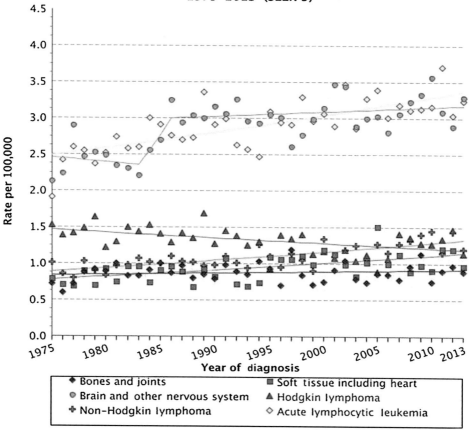

Age-adjusted SEER incidence rates
by cancer site
Ages < 20, all races, both sexes
1975–2013 (SEER 9)

Cancer sites include invasive cases only unless otherwise noted.
Rates are per 100,000 and are age-adjusted to the 2000 US Std Population (19 age groups – Census P25–1130). Regression lines are calculated using the Joinpoint Regression Program Version 4.2.0, April 2015, National Cancer Institute.
Incidence source: SEER 9 areas (San Francisco, Connecticut, Detroit, Hawaii, Iowa, New Mexico, Seattle, Utah, and Atlanta).

FIG. 1.7 Age-adjusted incidence rates by cancer site, United States, 1975–2013. (Data from Howlader N, Noone AM, Krapcho M, et al., eds. *SEER Cancer Statistics Review, 1975–2013*. Bethesda, MD: National Cancer Institute; April 2016. http://seer.cancer.gov/csr/1975_2013/, based on November 2015 SEER data submission, posted to the SEER web site.)

an average annual decrease of 0.6%. Other tumor types, including Wilm's tumor and malignant bone tumors, have remained steady over time (Fig. 1.7).

At this time, the cause of the increasing incidence rates in pediatric cancers overall remains unclear. Potential contributing factors include improved participation in cancer registries, improved access to medical care and diagnosis, and potential changes in environmental factors/exposures over time.

## MORTALITY RATES FOR CHILDHOOD AND ADOLESCENT CANCER

Death rates for pediatric and adolescent cancers have declined on an average of 2.1% per year since 1975. This has led to an overall decrease in the mortality rate for childhood cancer of over 50%.[5] Much of the decline in death rates for childhood cancer patients has been due to innovative multimodality therapies along with improvements in supportive care, such as central lines, antibiotics, and antifungal therapies. Despite these improvements, cancer remains the second leading cause of death for children, surpassed only by accidental deaths.[1] In 2014, there were an estimated 1350 deaths due to cancer in children aged 0–14 years, with an additional 610 cancer deaths expected in adolescents aged 15–19 years.[5] In addition, the average years of life lost per child (aged 0–14 years) dying of cancer is 71.8 years versus 19 years for persons dying of breast cancer and ~15 years for those who die of lung or colon cancer.[3]

The most marked improvements in death rates since the 1970's have been observed in patients treated for Hodgkin's lymphoma, acute lymphoblastic leukemia, and non-Hodgkin's lymphoma.[5] The distribution of disease-specific cancer deaths has remained fairly constant over time. In children aged 0–14 years, approximately one-third of the cancer deaths are due to leukemia, one-third are due to primary CNS malignancies, and the remaining one-third are mainly due to neuroblastoma, bone cancer, or sarcomas. In adolescents aged 15–19 years, leukemia remains the most common cause of cancer-related deaths, accounting for one-third of cases. This is followed by primary CNS malignancies (20%) and bone tumors (15%).[1]

Racial and ethnic disparities in the survival of pediatric cancer have been reported. For instance, although the incidence of cancer is lower in non-Hispanic blacks compared with whites and Hispanics, the death rates are similar. Researchers have suggested that the noted disparities may be multifactorial and related to socioeconomic status, parental education level, access to health insurance, time to diagnosis, participation in cooperative group trials, difference in disease biology, variations in adherence to prescribed therapies, and genetic polymorphisms involved in the metabolism of chemotherapeutic agents.[5]

## SURVIVAL RATES FOR CHILDHOOD AND ADOLESCENT CANCER

Since the 1950's survival rates for childhood and adolescent cancers have increased substantially. For a child diagnosed with cancer in the early 1950s the 5-year overall survival rate was 20%. For the period 2006–12, the 5-year survival rate for children diagnosed with cancer approached 85%.[3] As of January 1, 2011, there were 388,501 survivors of childhood cancer in the United States. Approximately 84% of those had survived 5 or more years from their original diagnosis, whereas 45% were alive 20 or more years from diagnosis.[8] As one

**TABLE 1.2**

**5-Year Relative Survival 1975–77 Versus 2006–12 by Selected Diagnosis for Ages 0–19 years**

| Diagnosis | 1975–77 | 2006–12 |
|---|---|---|
| Overall | 61.5 | 84.7 |
| Acute lymphoblastic leukemia | 53.8 | 91.0 |
| Acute myeloid leukemia | 18.7 | 66.2 |
| Hodgkin's lymphoma | 86.2 | 97.3 |
| Non-Hodgkin's lymphoma | 44.6 | 88.0 |
| Primary CNS malignancies | 58.9 | 75.1 |
| Neuroblastoma/ ganglioneuroblastoma | 53.1 | 76.8 |
| Wilm's (kidney tumors) | 72.6 | 92.6 |
| Soft tissue sarcomas | 64.8 | 78.2 |
| Bone cancer | 50.4 | 74.7 |

*CNS*, central nervous system; *SEER 18 areas*, San Francisco, Connecticut, Detroit, Hawaii, Iowa, New Mexico, Seattle, Utah, Atlanta, San Jose-Monterey, Los Angeles, Alaska Native Registry, Rural Georgia, California excluding SF/SJM/LA, Kentucky, Louisiana, New Jersey, and Georgia excluding ATL/RG.
Data from Howlader N, Noone AM, Krapcho M, et al., eds. *SEER Cancer Statistics Review, 1975–2013*. Bethesda, MD: National Cancer Institute; April 2016. http://seer.cancer.gov/csr/1975_2013/, based on November 2015 SEER data submission, posted to the SEER web site.

might expect from incidence rates, the cancer diagnosis with the largest number of survivors is leukemia, with 75,677 survivors as of 2011. This is followed by survivors of primary CNS malignancies (60,540), germ cell tumors (38,439), and renal tumors (23,990).[8] Table 1.2 compares 5-year survival rates from two eras (1975–77 vs. 2006–12) across select diagnostic groups.[3] Although marked improvements have been noted in many diagnostic groups, there are some childhood cancer diagnoses, such as bone cancers and soft tissue sarcomas, that still present significant challenges to achieving the goal of long-term cure.

Table 1.3 reports the 5-year relative survival rates by ICCC diagnosis during the period 2006–12 by sex for ages 0–19 years. Females seem to have a slightly increased survival rate in many disease categories when compared with males. Table 1.4 describes the 5-year survival percentages by ICCC diagnosis for both sexes, comparing childhood (ages 0–14 years) and adolescent patients (ages 15–19 years).[3] As noted in the table, for many cancer diagnoses, older age at

## TABLE 1.3
### 5 Year Relative Survival During 2006–12 by ICCC Diagnosis and Sex for Ages 0–19 years

| Diagnosis | Total Survival (%) | Male Survival (%) | Female Survival (%) |
|---|---|---|---|
| All groups | 83.3 | 82.1 | 84.6 |
| Leukemia—all | 83.3 | 82.8 | 83.4 |
| Acute lymphoblastic leukemia | 88.1 | 87.5 | 88.8 |
| Acute myeloid leukemia | 62.9 | 62.4 | 63.3 |
| Lymphoma—all | 93.1 | 92.9 | 93.2 |
| Hodgkin's lymphoma | 96.9 | 96.7 | 97.0 |
| Non-Hodgkin's lymphoma | 88.8 | 89.3 | 87.7 |
| Primary CNS malignancies | 73.8 | 72.9 | 74.8 |
| Ependymoma/choroid plexus tumors | 77.9 | 77.3 | 78.6 |
| Astrocytoma | 82.6 | 81.1 | 84.1 |
| Embryonal tumors | 62.8 | 62.3 | 63.5 |
| Other gliomas | 59.9 | 63.4 | 56.2 |
| Neuroblastoma/ganglioneuroblastoma | 79.5 | 78 | 81.2 |
| Retinoblastoma | 95.3 | 94.2 | 96.5 |
| Kidney tumors | 89.2 | 87.2 | 91.1 |
| Nephroblastoma | 91.1 | 89.3 | 92.8 |
| Hepatic tumors | 72.4 | 71,3 | 74.6 |
| Hepatoblastoma | 83.9 | 82 | 87.9 |
| Malignant bone tumors | 70.7 | 69.1 | 73.0 |
| Osteosarcoma | 67 | 65.1 | 69.4 |
| Ewing's sarcoma | 71.7 | 68.8 | 76.9 |
| Soft tissue sarcomas | 72.3 | 70.5 | 74.5 |
| Rhabdomyosarcoma | 65.8 | 66.5 | 64.9 |
| Germ cell tumors | 92.4 | 92.8 | 91.6 |
| intracranial/intraspinal | 90 | 91.1 | 85.6 |
| gonadal | 96.7 | 96.1 | 97.8 |
| Malignant melanoma | 93.9 | 91.1 | 96.0 |
| Thyroid carcinoma | 99.7 | 98.9 | 99.8 |

CNS, central nervous system; ICCC, International Classification of Childhood Cancer; SEER 18 areas, San Francisco, Connecticut, Detroit, Hawaii, Iowa, New Mexico, Seattle, Utah, Atlanta, San Jose-Monterey, Los Angeles, Alaska Native Registry, Rural Georgia, California excluding SF/SJM/LA, Kentucky, Louisiana, New Jersey, and Georgia excluding ATL/RG.
Based on Surveillance, Epidemiology and End Results Program data from Howlader N, Noone AM, Krapcho M, et al., eds. SEER Cancer Statistics Review, 1975–2013. Bethesda, MD: National Cancer Institute; April 2016. http://seer.cancer.gov/csr/1975_2013/, based on November 2015 SEER data submission, posted to the SEER web site.

diagnosis is a poor prognostic sign and is associated with decreased survival percentages. There is much attention at this time to the worse outcomes seen in the AYA (adolescent and young adult) population and many factors may be influential, including less favorable biologic features of their cancer, decreased participation in cooperative group trials, and health insurance status.[9] Finally, based on SEER data from 2003 to 2009, non-Hispanic white children and adolescents diagnosed with cancer have improved survival percentages compared with non-Hispanic black and Hispanic populations.

As the overall 5-year survival rate for children and adolescents diagnosed with cancer stands now at 85%, there has been increased interest in and emphasis on the long-term complications those survivors may face due to their original cancer diagnosis and treatment. As Phillips et al. stated, "a singular focus on curing cancer

**TABLE 1.4**

**5-Year Relative Survival During 2006–12 for Both Sexes by ICCC Diagnosis and Age at Diagnosis**

| By ICCC Subgroup | <1 year | 1–4 year | 5–9 year | 10–14 year | 15–19 year | 0–14 year |
|---|---|---|---|---|---|---|
| All groups | 78.7 | 84.5 | 83.2 | 82.3 | 83.9 | 83.0 |
| Leukemia—all | 62.0 | 90.0 | 89.3 | 77.8 | 71.3 | 85.6 |
|   Acute lymphoblastic leukemia | 60.8 | 93.7 | 92.6 | 82.2 | 74.7 | 90.2 |
|   Acute myeloid leukemia | 60.0 | 66.5 | 69.1 | 61.2 | 59.7 | 64.2 |
| Lymphoma—all | 79.9 | 92.6 | 94.1 | 93.8 | 92.7 | 93.4 |
|   Hodgkin's lymphoma | – | 94.5 | 97.7 | 97.9 | 96.4 | 97.7 |
|   Non-Hodgkin's lymphoma | – | 91.3 | 92.2 | 89.7 | 86.0 | 90.7 |
| Primary CNS malignancies | 60.3 | 72.8 | 70.6 | 78.6 | 79.1 | 72.6 |
|   Ependymoma/choroid plexus tumors | 65.3 | 74.7 | 77.5 | 82.1 | 88.1 | 75.9 |
|   Astrocytoma | 81.8 | 90.6 | 80.5 | 81.3 | 77.2 | 83.9 |
|   Embryonal tumors | 29.1 | 55.6 | 70.6 | 76.8 | 73.2 | 61.5 |
|   Other gliomas | – | 49.2 | 44.7 | 70.4 | 83.3 | 54.1 |
| Neuroblastoma/ganglioneuroblastoma | 93.8 | 73.8 | 70.2 | 72.3 | 74.2 | 79.7 |
| Retinoblastoma | 97.0 | 93.5 | – | – | – | 95.3 |
| Kidney tumors | 94.0 | 91.0 | 90.1 | 76.3 | 68.1 | 90.6 |
|   Nephroblastoma | 94.0 | 91.2 | 91.7 | 82.1 | – | 91.5 |
| Hepatic tumors | 86.3 | 83.1 | 67.5 | 35.4 | 47.4 | 77.1 |
|   Hepatoblastoma | 85.9 | 83.1 | – | – | – | 84.2 |
| Malignant bone tumors | – | 80.2 | 77.6 | 72.2 | 65.7 | 74.2 |
|   Osteosarcoma | – | – | 72.4 | 68.8 | 63.4 | 69.5 |
|   Ewing's sarcoma | – | 94.6 | 83.0 | 72.9 | 59.2 | 78.7 |
| Soft tissue sarcoma | 64.5 | 75.8 | 78.8 | 72.6 | 69.1 | 74.0 |
|   Rhabdomyosarcoma | 53.0 | 72.7 | 78.7 | 59.2 | 48.9 | 69.6 |
| Germ cell tumors | 87.7 | 93.3 | 98.3 | 94.0 | 91.9 | 93.9 |
|   Intracranial/intraspinal | – | – | 98.4 | 91.1 | 89.2 | 90.4 |
|   Gonadal | 100 | 100 | 98.0 | 99.4 | 95.7 | 99.4 |
| Malignant melanoma | – | 96.3 | 96.0 | 94.2 | 94.0 | 93.7 |
| Thyroid carcinoma | – | – | 98.1 | 100 | 99.7 | 99.7 |

CNS, central nervous system; ICCC, International Classification of Childhood Cancer; SEER 18 areas, San Francisco, Connecticut, Detroit, Hawaii, Iowa, New Mexico, Seattle, Utah, Atlanta, San Jose-Monterey, Los Angeles, Alaska Native Registry, Rural Georgia, California excluding SF/SJM/LA, Kentucky, Louisiana, New Jersey, and Georgia excluding ATL/RG.
Based on Surveillance, Epidemiology and End Results Program data from Howlader N, Noone AM, Krapcho M, et al., eds. SEER Cancer Statistics Review, 1975–2013. Bethesda, MD: National Cancer Institute; April 2016. http://seer.cancer.gov/csr/1975_2013/, based on November 2015 SEER data submission, posted to the SEER web site.

yields an incomplete picture of childhood cancer survivors" because the burden of chronic conditions faced by this population is profound both in its occurrence and severity.[8]

## CHILDHOOD CANCER SURVIVORSHIP

The improvement in survival rates in childhood and adolescent cancer is due to many factors, most notably advances in multimodality therapies, improved risk stratification, optimizing supportive care, and participation in cooperative group studies. However, this improvement does not come without cost. Survivors of childhood cancer are at increased risk of many adverse health or quality-of-life outcomes, including increased incidence and severity of chronic health conditions, health limitations, frequent hospitalizations, premature frailty, psychologic distress, neurocognitive dysfunction, and decreased productivity.[8,10–13] Development of complications of therapy is dependent on many factors, including the type and cumulative dose of chemotherapeutic agents, age at therapy, family history, lifestyle practices, and exposure to ionizing radiation.[14] The Childhood Cancer Survivor Study (CCSS) is a cohort study that follows childhood cancer survivors in North America who were diagnosed at less than 21 years of age, are alive with one of eight major cancer subtypes, and survived at least 5 years from original diagnosis. It combined detailed medical record abstraction with patient questionnaires and has contributed much to the field of childhood cancer survivorship.[15]

A study by the CCSS examined late mortality in ~20,000 childhood cancer survivors and found that they had 8.4 times higher mortality rate than age- and sex-matched peers in the general population of the United States. The highest mortality rate was in the first 5 years on entering the cohort, when the risk of recurrence was highest. However, their risk for death remains substantially elevated, and by 15 years after diagnosis the main cause of death is due to secondary malignancies.[16] Oeffinger et al. again, using the CCSS population, found that an estimated 68% of childhood cancer survivors have at least one chronic health condition 5–14 years after diagnosis, with one-third of survivors reporting severe or life-threatening chronic conditions. The prevalence of chronic conditions in this population continues to increase as they age; by 15–24 years postdiagnosis 77% of survivors report at least one chronic condition and 85% are affected 25–36 years postdiagnosis.[17]

Survivors of childhood cancer are at an estimated three- to sixfold increased risk of developing subsequent primary neoplasms compared with the general population. The CCSS found a 20-year cumulative incidence of 3.2% for secondary neoplasms and this increased to 9.3% by 30 years from diagnosis.[18] The British CCSS cohort explored the incidence of subsequent cancers in an older population and found that excess risk still exists even 40 years after diagnosis.[19] The largest excess risk for childhood cancer survivors was seen for the following subsequent neoplasms: breast cancer (standardized incidence ratio [SIR] of 16.2), bone cancer (SIR 19.1), and thyroid cancer (SIR 11.3). Female survivors treated with chest radiation have a markedly elevated risk of developing breast cancer with a SIR of 24.7.[18] Survivors treated with radiation to the abdomen and/or pelvis were found to have a comparable risk of developing colorectal cancer as an individual with two or more first-degree relatives affected by colorectal cancer.[19] Analyses have identified many risk factors for the

development of subsequent cancers including female gender, younger age at original diagnosis, exposure to certain chemotherapy drugs at increased doses (alkylating agents, anthracyclines, and epipodophyllotoxins), exposure to radiotherapy, and a primary diagnosis of Hodgkin's lymphoma, bone cancer, or soft tissue sarcoma.[18,19] Much effort is being focused on understanding the role genetics may play in the development of secondary cancers in childhood cancer survivors. An analysis of the family history in survivors who went on to develop secondary neoplasms found an elevated risk of cancer in siblings when compared with the general population.[18,20]

## RISK FACTORS FOR PEDIATRIC MALIGNANCY

Over the last several decades, many studies have sought to identify possible causes and risk factors for pediatric malignancy. However, identifying causes and risk factors for pediatric malignancy is difficult given the rarity of childhood cancer. Because the overall incidence of pediatric malignancy is low, most studies of potential extrinsic risk factors rely on case-control study designs, which have inherent weaknesses of recall and selection bias that may compromise the quality of the data. In addition, the rarity of pediatric malignancy means that data accumulate slowly, and it is only in the most common pediatric malignancies, acute leukemias, and CNS tumors that enough data have accumulated to allow for metaanalysis. However, metaanalysis is also limited by the biases of the primary research, by what is reported or not reported by the primary researcher, and by the clinical diversity and varying characteristics of the trials used in the metaanalysis. The heterogeneity of pediatric cancer also makes identifying causes and risk factors more difficult because different types of malignancy likely have different combinations of factors that contribute to their development. It is likely that pediatric malignancies, like adult malignancies, are caused by a combination of genetic and environmental factors, and it may be difficult to determine how much of a role any one particular factor may play in the development of pediatric malignancy. It is important to consider all of these potential limitations when critically evaluating the literature available on risk factors for pediatric malignancy.

Demographic risk factor for pediatric maligancy were discussed previously in the Pediatric Cancer Incidence by Age and Cancer Type, Pediatric Cancer Incidence by Gender, and Pediatric Cancer Incidence by

Race/Ethnicity sections of this chapter. Other risk factors can be divided into environmental risk factors, intrinsic risk factors, and genetic risk factors.

## ENVIRONMENTAL/EXTRINSIC RISK FACTORS

Extrinsic or environmental risk factors are those factors or exposure that arise from outside the patient's body. Multiple studies have been done over the years to elucidate possible environmental or external causes of pediatric malignancy. Well-established data exist to support prior chemotherapy and exposure to ionizing radiation as extrinsic causes of pediatric malignancy, and these are widely accepted as contributing factors to development of pediatric malignancy in the scientific community. Data regarding other possible extrinsic or environmental factors are less well established, and there may be conflicting results among studies. As mentioned previously, many studies evaluating extrinsic factors are case-control or metaanalysis designs, which have inherent weaknesses and biases. In addition, environmental factors that could influence development of childhood cancers require being separated into maternal exposures before the onset of pregnancy, exposure during pregnancy, and exposure that occur postnatal. These limitations in study design and data collection make establishing a definitive causal relationship between an extrinsic factor and pediatric malignancy difficult.

### Chemotherapy

Although great strides have been made in the cure rate and survival of pediatric patients with malignancy through the use of multiagent chemotherapy regimens, a potential consequence of this success is the increased risk of secondary malignancies. Particular chemotherapies, including alkylating agents and topoisomerase inhibitors, have been identified as causes of secondary malignancies in pediatric patients, most commonly treatment-related acute myelogenous leukemia.[16,21-27] The cancer-causing effect of these chemotherapy medications is related to direct DNA damage in normal cells caused by the drug.

Common alkylating agents used in the treatment of pediatric malignancies include cyclophosphamide, ifosfamide, melphalan, busulfan, and cisplatin, among several others. Alkylating agents are commonly used in the treatment of pediatric leukemias, lymphomas, and sarcomas. Reports from the CCSS found that exposure to alkylating agents during treatment for a pediatric malignancy resulted in a relative risk (RR) of

mortality from secondary malignancy of 1.4–2.2 with a dose-response relationship seen as patients with higher total alkylating agent dose exposure having increased RR compared with those at lower doses.[16] The risk of treatment-related leukemia, most commonly acute myelogenous leukemia, as a result of exposure to alkylating agents is particularly high, with an RR of 4.8.[21] Again, a strong dose-response relationship was observed between leukemia risk and total dose of alkylating agents. The treatment-related acute myelogenous leukemia (AML) arising from alkylating agent exposure has specific cytogenetic abnormalities, including monosomy or partial deletions of chromosome 5 and 7, and typically occur in a time frame of 5–7 years after treatment.[22-24]

Topoisomerase inhibitors, which include both anthracyclines and epipodophyllotoxins, have also been shown to increase the risk of secondary malignancy in pediatric patients treated for malignancy. Like alkylating agents, topoisomerase inhibitors are classically associated with causing treatment-related acute myelogenous leukemia.[25] The incidence rates of secondary leukemia after treatment with a topoisomerase inhibitor varies in the literature but has been reported as high as 8.3%.[26] In the CCSS, the RR of mortality from secondary malignancy after treatment with an epipodophyllotoxin was up to 2.3 in those patients with the highest total dose exposure.[16] The same study showed an RR of mortality from secondary malignancy of 1.4 in patients with the highest total dose exposure to anthracyclines as well. Treatment-related AML secondary to epipodophyllotoxins is classically associated with the mixed lineage leukemia (MLL) gene rearrangement (11q23).[27] Treatment-related AML associated with both anthracyclines and epipodophyllotoxins typically appears more acutely, with an onset within 2–3 years of treatment.[24]

### Ionizing Radiation

Ionizing radiation is high-energy particles that result in freeing of electrons from molecules as they pass through the molecule, causing ionization. Ionizing radiation passing through human tissue can lead to DNA damage, either directly or through the generation of free radicals. When DNA damage is double-stranded, it is more difficult to repair and this can ultimately contribute to the development of malignancy. Studies in atomic bomb survivors show that there is an increased risk of leukemia and solid tumors resulting from the exposure to ionizing radiation, and studies show that patients who have undergone ionizing radiation treatment for primary malignancy are also at increased risk of secondary malignancies.[16,24,28,29] There is also increasing evidence suggesting a link between repeated low-dose radiation exposure from diagnostic imaging techniques, such as X-ray, fluoroscopy and computed-tomography (CT) scans, and the development of malignancy later in life. Data also suggest that younger children are more sensitive to the effects of radiation than adults, and as children they also have a longer lifetime during which malignancy could develop as the result of the exposure to ionizing radiation.[30–33]

A significant amount of the information available linking ionizing radiation exposure and subsequent development of malignancies arises from survivors of the atomic bombs in Japan, through the Life Span Study (LSS).[28] The LSS is a large cohort of atomic bomb survivors who have been followed since the start of the 1950s and has made a substantial contribution to the understanding of the effect of ionizing radiation exposure on humans. In the LSS, excess cases of leukemia were reported as early as 3 years from the time of the bombings and the risk of leukemia among survivors increased in the 6–8 years after the bombings. Children who were around age 10 years at the time of exposure were found to have a peak excess RR of leukemia of 70 that rapidly declined to 1–3 with increasing time from exposure, whereas those who were exposed at age 30 years or older had an excess RR of 2 throughout the time since exposure to the bombing. In addition to leukemias, increased risk of solid malignancies was seen in the LSS, beginning ~10 years from the time of the bombings. Again, the excess RR of solid malignancies was higher in those exposed during childhood than during adults. The increased risk of both leukemia and solid malignancies seen in pediatric survivors of the atomic bomb compared with adult survivors suggests children are inherently more sensitive to the effects of ionizing radiation exposure.

Ionizing radiation also plays an integral part in the treatment of many malignancies, including pediatric malignancies such as CNS tumors, solid tumors, Hodgkin's lymphoma, and leukemias, and in the conditioning regimen for hematopoietic stem cell transplant. In the CCSS, radiation exposure during treatment for pediatric malignancy resulted in an RR of mortality from secondary malignancy of 2.9,[16] and treatment with ionizing radiation was the strongest independent risk factor for the development of second malignant neoplasm in survivors of pediatric malignancies.[29] The typical time to development of a secondary malignancy after exposure to ionizing radiation used for the treatment of pediatric malignancy is approximately 10–15 years.[24] The most common secondary malignancies seen in children with prior ionizing radiation included nonmelanoma skin cancer, breast and thyroid cancer, bone tumors, and benign CNS tumors, such as meningiomas.[24]

Although the data are less strong than for high-dose exposure such as the atomic bombs or treatment dose exposure to ionizing radiation, there is increasing concern that repeated low-dose ionizing radiation exposure may increase the risk of malignancy in children and adolescents later in life. With the increasing use of diagnostic imaging, such as CT scans and fluoroscopy, diagnostic radiation now accounts for ~50% of the total radiation exposure of the US population.[33] One recent retrospective cohort study of pediatric cancer patients with leukemias and malignant brain tumors from the United Kingdom revealed that patients who received higher cumulative doses of ionizing radiation were at a 3.2 times greater risk of developing a subsequent leukemia and at a 2.8 times greater risk of developing subsequent brain tumors.[34] However, the absolute risk remained extremely small, with only one excess case of leukemia and one excess case of brain tumor for every 10,000 CT scans. A study from Australia that included ~11 million individuals has found a statistically significant positive association between CT scan exposure and brain tumor development. The risk of brain tumor development in this study was inversely related to increasing age at the time of first exposure to CT scan radiation, increasing years since the first exposure, and increasing calendar year of the first exposure.[32] An additional retrospective cohort study from the United States evaluating the use of diagnostic CT scans and cancer risks in the pediatric population reported an increased projected lifetime attributable risk of solid cancer in younger patients and females when compared with older patients and males. This study also found that the risk of leukemia from head CT scans was highest with a rate of 1.9 cases per 10,000 CTs. Based on the national average of 4 million CT scans of the head, chest, abdomen/pelvis, or spine each year, the study projected that nearly 4900 cases of future cancer were caused by CT each year.[33]

### Other Environmental/Extrinsic Exposures

Outside of prior chemotherapy and ionizing radiation, no other environmental or extrinsic exposures are widely accepted to have a causative association with pediatric malignancy, although positive and negative correlations have been found to suggest potential relationships between certain exposures and development of pediatric malignancy. Among those extrinsic factors that have been evaluated are exposure to infections (mainly indirect measure of infectious exposure such

**TABLE 1.5**
Results of Selected Metaanalyses of Associations Between Extrinsic Risk Factors and Pediatric Acute Lymphoblastic Leukemia (ALL)

| Exposure | Timing of Exposure | Findings | References |
|---|---|---|---|
| Maternal prenatal vitamins | Pregnancy | Decreased risk of ALL with maternal prenatal vitamin supplementation. mOR 0.61(95% CI 0.50–0.74) | 34 |
| Pesticide exposure | Pregnancy | Increased risk of pediatric ALL with maternal occupational exposure to pesticides during pregnancy. mOR 2.64 (95% CI 1.40–5.00) | 35 |
|  | Postnatal | Increased risk of pediatric ALL with exposure to indoor pesticides during childhood. mOR 1.47 (95% CI 1.26–1.72). No association with outdoor pesticide exposure | 36 |
| Maternal smoking | Pregnancy | No association between maternal smoking during pregnancy and pediatric ALL. mOR 1.03 (95% CI 0.95–1.12) | 37 |
| Maternal alcohol | Pregnancy | No association between maternal alcohol intake during pregnancy and pediatric ALL. mOR 1.10 (95% CI 0.93–1.29) | 38 |
| Infectious exposures | Postnatal | Decreased risk of ALL in children who attended day care. mOR 0.76 (95% CI 0.67–0.87) | 39 |
| Nonionizing radiation | Postnatal | No association between electromagnetic field exposure and pediatric ALL. mOR 1.25 (95% CI 0.97–1.60) | 40 |

CI, confidence interval; mOR, metaanalytic odds ratio.

as day-care attendance), residential and maternal occupational pesticide exposure, maternal alcohol, smoking, and vitamin use. The majority of these data exist in pediatric acute lymphoblastic leukemia (ALL) and pediatric brain tumors, as these are the most common malignancies in childhood and allow for the highest number of patients to evaluate for potential exposures. Results of recent metaanalyses of extrinsic exposures and pediatric ALL are presented in Table 1.5. Results of recent case-control studies and metaanalyses evaluating the relationship between pediatric brain tumors and extrinsic exposures are presented in Table 1.6.

Regarding maternal medication use, a small decrease in the risk of pediatric ALL was seen with maternal prenatal vitamin exposure, but no similar association was seen in PBTs.[34,41,42] Parental occupation exposure to pesticides does show a positive association with the development of both pediatric ALL and PBTs.[35,43,44] In addition, residential exposure to pesticides was found to have a positive association with pediatric ALL.[36] Day-care attendance, as an indirect measurement of infectious exposure, was found to lead to a decreased risk

of both pediatric ALL and PBTs.[39,48] No other environmental exposures have been found to have significant associations with either pediatric ALL or PBTs, including maternal alcohol use or smoking and nonionizing forms of radiation exposure.

## INTRINSIC RISK FACTORS
Intrinsic risk factors are those that are inherent to the person and not from an external source. Several intrinsic risk factors have been shown to be associated with increased risk of childhood malignancies. These factors include birthweight and maternal age.

Birthweight has been shown in several studies to be associated with increased risk of certain pediatric malignancies. A recent large case-control study using population-based data sets from both the United States and the United Kingdom found that many childhood cancers show a positive association with increasing birthweight, many exhibiting a linear relationship between increasing birthweight and increasing risk of childhood malignancies.[53] These malignancies included ALL, renal tumors

**TABLE 1.6**
**Results of Selected Studies Evaluating Associations Between Environmental Exposures and Pediatric Brain Tumors (PBTs)**

| Exposure | Timing of Exposure | Findings | References |
|---|---|---|---|
| Maternal medications | Pregnancy | No significant associations between maternally reported medications and PBTs. Medications evaluated included diuretics/antihypertensives, pain relievers, antiemetics, and cold medications. Case-control study | 41 |
| | | No significant associations found for antacids, laxatives, iron, folic acid, diuretics, antibiotics, analgesics, antiemetics, antihistamines, neuroleptics, and antiasthma tics. However, positive association was found with β-blocker antihypertensives (OR 5.3, 95% CI 1.2–24.8). Linkage study | 42 |
| Pesticide exposure | Prenatal | Significant positive association between PBTs and paternal but not maternal occupational pesticide exposure. OR for paternal exposure 1.4 (95% CI 1.20–1.62). Metaanalysis | 43 |
| | | Significant positive association between parents with prenatal occupational pesticide exposure and PBTs. Summary OR 1.30 (95% CI 1.11–1.53). Metaanalysis | 44 |
| Maternal smoking | Pregnancy | No association between maternal tobacco exposure and PBTs. Metaanalysis | 45 |
| Maternal alcohol | Pregnancy | No association between alcohol exposure in utero and risk for PBTs. Case-control | 46 |
| Infectious exposures | Postnatal | Increased risk of PBTs in children with no social exposure to other infants in the first year of life. OR 1.37 (95% CI 1.08–1.75). Case-control | 47 |
| | | Decreased risk of PBTs in children who attended day care for > 1 year or were breast-fed. Case-control | 48 |
| | | No association between breast-feeding and PBTs | 49 |
| Nonionizing radiation | Postnatal | No association between residential AM-radio transmission and PBTs. Case-control | 50 |
| | | No association between residential magnetic field exposure and PBTs. Metaanalysis | 51 |
| | | No association between cell phone use in 7- to 19-year-olds and PBTs. Case-control | 52 |

*OR*, odds ratio.

(excluding Wilm's tumor), CNS tumors, soft tissue sarcomas, neuroblastoma, lymphomas, and non-CNS germ cell tumors. Risk for other tumor types showed an association with birthweight but in a nonlinear fashion, including AML, Wilm's tumor, and hepatoblastoma. For AML, there was a U-shaped relationship with increased risk seen in both low- and high-birthweight infants. Wilm's tumor was found to be associated with only high birthweights, and hepatoblastoma was found to have a high correlation with very low birthweights. These findings are consistent with prior studies looking at the risk of pediatric malignancies and birthweight.[54–60] The biologic mechanism explaining the association between increased birthweight and malignancy has not been elucidated or well studied, but potential explanations included increased exposure to prenatal growth factors, such as insulin-like growth factor,[61] and the increased number of cells at risk for malignant transformation.[53] For hepatoblastoma, where there is a significantly increased risk in the very premature and very low birthweight infants, there is some thought that the medications and treatments administered to the very premature infant may have carcinogenic effects on the liver. However, no particular treatment or medication has been identified as the causative agent.[62]

Advanced parental age has been associated with several diseases in childhood, including congenital syndromes that can be predisposed to cancer. Because of this, several studies have been done to evaluate if increasing parental age can contribute to childhood cancer development. Most studies have been inconsistent.[63,64] However, a large case-control study using pooled population-based data did show a positive linear trend per 5-year increase in maternal age for risk of childhood cancer overall and in 7 out of 10 of the most common pediatric diagnosis.[65] Positive trends were seen for leukemia, lymphoma, CNS tumors, neuroblastoma, Wilm's tumor, bone tumors, and soft tissue sarcomas. No maternal age association was seen in germ cell tumors, hepatoblastoma, or retinoblastoma. When controlling for maternal age, no association was seen with advancing paternal age and risk of childhood malignancy. However, maternal and paternal age are highly correlated; therefore it may be difficult to determine if it is solely maternal age that contributes to the increased risk of childhood malignancy or if paternal age is playing a role as well. The biologic mechanism to explain the link between advancing maternal age and increased risk of childhood malignancies has not been elucidated to date.

## GENETIC RISK FACTORS

Inherited syndromes are known to cause a small minority of childhood cancer cases. Traditionally, it is estimated that 5%–10% of cases of childhood malignancy can be attributed to inherited cancer predisposition syndromes.[66,67] However, this number is difficult to quantify because there are likely cases that go unidentified, particularly if a genetic mutation arises de novo and there is no suspicious family history that leads to further evaluation and testing. In addition, there are specific tumor types, such as retinoblastoma and adrenocortical carcinoma, where the fraction of cases caused by a genetic predisposition syndrome are much higher. Cancer predisposition syndromes can be grouped into one of three types of genes: tumor suppressor genes, oncogenes, and DNA stability genes.[68] There are currently numerous inherited cancer predisposition syndromes that have been well defined to cause malignancy in the pediatric age group and this list is steadily growing as our knowledge of the human genome continues to increase. Table 1.7 includes a brief summary of the most common inherited cancer predisposition syndromes and these syndromes will be discussed in more detail in later chapters of this book. The study of the families affected by genetic cancer predisposition syndromes is of great value in understanding the development of certain pediatric malignancies as the genes found to be mutated in these syndromes are also found as somatic mutations within sporadic cancers.

**TABLE 1.7**
**Inherited Cancer Predisposition Syndromes**

| Syndrome | Gene | Gene Type | Mode of Inheritance | Tumor Types |
|---|---|---|---|---|
| **CENTRAL NERVOUS SYSTEM PREDISPOSITION SYNDROMES** | | | | |
| Retinoblastoma | RBI | TS | AD | Retinoblastoma, osteosarcoma |
| Rhabdoid predisposition syndrome | SNF5/INI1 | TS | UC | ATRT, rhabdoid tumor of kidney, medulloblastoma, choroid plexus tumor |
| Medulloblastoma predisposition | SUFU | TS | AD | Medulloblastoma |
| **GASTROINTESTINAL MALIGNANCY PREDISPOSITION SYNDROMES** | | | | |
| Adenomatous polyposis of the colon | APC | TS | AD | Colon, thyroid, stomach, intestine, hepatoblastoma |
| Juvenile polyposis | SMAD4/DP C4 | TS | AD | Gastrointestinal |
| Peutz-Jeghers syndrome | STKII | TS | AD | Intestinal, ovarian, pancreatic |

**TABLE 1.7**
Inherited Cancer Predisposition Syndromes—cont'd

| Syndrome | Gene | Gene Type | Mode of Inheritance | Tumor Types |
|---|---|---|---|---|
| **ENDOCRINE CANCER PREDISPOSITION SYNDROMES** | | | | |
| Hereditary paraganglioma and pheochromocytoma syndrome | SOH | TS | AD/paternal | Paragangliomas, pheochromocytomas |
| MENI | MENI | TS | AD | Pancreatic islet cell tumor, pituitary adenoma, parathyroid adenoma |
| MEN2 | RET | OG | AD | Medullary thyroid carcinoma, pheochromocytoma, parathyroid hyperplasia |
| **GENITOURINARY CANCER PREDISPOSITION SYNDROMES** | | | | |
| Beckwith-Wiedemann syndrome | CDKNIC/N SOI | TS | AD | Wilm's tumor, hepatoblastoma, adrenal carcinoma, rhabdomyosarcoma |
| DICERI syndrome | DICERI | TS | AD | Pleuropulmonary blastoma, ovarian sertoli-Leydig cell tumors, cystic nephroma, embryonal rhabdomyosarcoma, multinodular goiter |
| Von Hippel-Lindau syndrome | VHL | TS | AD | Hemangioblastomas, pheochromocytoma, renal cell carcinoma |
| WAGR syndrome | WTI | TS | AD | Wilm's tumor, gonadoblastoma |
| Wilm's tumor syndrome | WTI | TS | AD | Wilm's tumor |
| **GENODERMATOSES WITH CANCER PREDISPOSITION** | | | | |
| Nevoid basal cell carcinoma syndrome | PTCH | TS | AD | Skin, medulloblastoma |
| Neurofibromatosis type 1 | Nfl | TS | AD | Neurofibroma, optic pathway glioma, peripheral nerve sheath tumor |
| Neurofibromatosis type 2 | NF2 | TS | AD | Vestibular schwannoma |
| Rothmund-Thomson Syndrome | RECQL4 | SG | AR | Skin, bone |
| Tuberous sclerosis | TSC1/TSC2 | TS | AD | Hamartoma, renal angiomyolipoma, renal cell carcinoma |
| Xeroderma pigmentosum | XP,POLH | SG | AR | Skin, melanoma, leukemia |
| **LEUKEMIA/LYMPHOMA PREDISPOSITION SYNDROMES** | | | | |
| Ataxia telangiectasia | ATM | SG | AR | Leukemia, lymphoma |
| Bloom syndrome | BLM | SG | AR | Leukemia, lymphoma, skin |
| Fanmni anemia | FANC | SG | AR | Leukemia, squamous cell carcinoma |
| Nijmegen breakage syndrome | NBSI | SG | AR | Lymphoma, medulloblastoma, glioma |

*Continued*

**TABLE 1.7**
Inherited Cancer Predisposition Syndromes—cont'd

| Syndrome | Gene | Gene Type | Mode of Inheritance | Tumor Types |
|---|---|---|---|---|
| **SARCOMA CANCER PREDISPOSITION SYNDROMES** | | | | |
| Li-Fraumeni syndrome | TP53 | TS | AD | Soft tissue sarcoma, osteosarcoma, breast adrenocorticocarcinoma, leukemia, choroid plexus carcinoma |
| Multiple exotosis | EXT1/EXT2 | TS | AD | Chondrosarcoma |
| Werner syndrome | WRN | SG | AR | Osteosarcoma, meningioma |

*AD*, autosomal dominant; *AR*, autosomal recessive; *OG*, oncogene; *SG*, stability gene; *TS*, tumor suppressor gene; *UC*, unclear.

## REFERENCES

1. Scheurer ME, Lupo PJ, Bondy ML. Epidemiology of childhood cancer. In: Pizzo PA, Poplack DG, eds. *Principles and Practice of Pediatric Oncology*. 7th ed. Philadelphia, PA: Lippincott, Williams, and Wilkins; 2015:1–5.
2. Steliarova-Foucher E, Stiller C, Lacour B, Kaatsch P. International classification of childhood cancer- third edition. *Cancer*. 2005;103:1457–1567.
3. Howlader N, Noone AM, Krapcho M, et al., eds. *SEER Cancer Statistics Review, 1975-2013*. Bethesda, MD: National Cancer Institute; April 2016. Based on November 2015 SEER data submission, posted to the SEER web site. http://seer.cancer.gov/csr/1975_2013/.
4. Copeland G, Lake A, Firth R, et al. Cancer in North America: 2008-2012. In: *Combined Cancer Incidence for the United States, Canada and North America*. Vol. 1. Springfield, IL: North American Association of Central Cancer Registries Inc; 2015.
5. Ward E, Desantis C, Robbins A, Kohler B, Jemal A. Childhood and adolescent cancer statistics, 2014. *CA Cancer J Clin*. 2014;64:83–103.
6. Spector LG, Ross JA, Olshan AF. Children's oncology group 2013 blueprint for research: epidemiology. *Pediatr Blood Cancer*. 2013;60:1059–1062.
7. Last JM, ed. *Dictionary of Epidemiology*. 4th ed. New York: Oxford University Press; 2001:61.
8. Phillips SM, Padgett LS, Leisenring W, et al. Survivors of childhood cancer in the United States: prevalence and burden of morbidity. *Cancer Epidemiol Biomarkers Prev*. 2015;24(4):653–663.
9. Freyer DR, Felgenhauer J, Perentesis J. Children's oncology group 2013 blueprint for research: adolescent and young adult oncology. *Pediatr Blood Cancer*. 2013;60:1055–1058.
10. Hudson MM, Mertens AC, Yasui Y, et al. Health status of adult long-term survivors of childhood cancer: a report from the Childhood Cancer Survivor Study. *JAMA*. 2003;290(12):1583–1592.
11. Dowling E, Yabroff KR, Mariotto A. Burden of illness in adult survivors of childhood cancer. *Cancer*. 2010;116(15):3712–3721.
12. Hoffman MC, Mulrooney DA, Steinberger J, et al. Deficits in physical function among young childhood cancer survivors. *J Clin Oncol*. 2013;31:2799–2805.
13. Zhang Y, Lorenzi MF, Goddard K. Late morbidity leading to hospitalization among 5 year survivors of young adult cancer: a report of the childhood, adolescent, and young adult cancer survivors research program. *Int J Cancer*. 2014;134:1174–1182.
14. Landier W, Bhatia S, Eshelman D, et al. Development of risk based guidelines for pediatric cancer survivors: The Children's Oncology Group Long-Term Follow-Up Guidelines from the Children's Oncology Group Late Effects Committee and Nursing Discipline. *J Clin Oncol*. 2004;22:4979–4990.
15. Robinson LL, Mertens AC, Boice JD, et al. Study design and cohort characteristics of the Childhood Cancer Survivor Study: a multi-institutional collaborative project. *Med Pediatr Oncol*. 2002;38(4):229–239.
16. Mertens AC, Lui Q, Neglia JP, et al. Cause-specific late mortality among 5-year survivors of childhood cancer: the Childhood Cancer Survivor Study. *J Natl Cancer Inst*. 2008;100(19):1368–1379.
17. Oeffinger KC, Mertens AC, Sklar CA, et al. Chronic health conditions in adult survivors of childhood cancer. *New Engl J Med*. 2006;355(15):1572–1582.
18. Meadows AT, Friedman DL, Neglia JP, et al. Second neoplasms in survivors of childhood cancer: findings from the childhood cancer survivor study. *J Clin Oncol*. 2009;27:2356–2362.
19. Reulen RC, Frobisher C, Winter DL, et al. Longterm risks of subsequent primary neoplasms among survivors of childhood cancers. *JAMA*. 2011;305(22):2311–2319.
20. Friedman DL, Kadan-Lottick N, Whitton J, et al. Increased risk of cancer among siblings of long-term childhood cancer survivors: a report from the childhood cancer survivor study. *Cancer Epidemiol Biomarkers Prev*. 2005;14(8):1922–1927.
21. Tucker MA, Meadows AT, Boice Jr JD, et al. Leukemia after therapy with alkylating agents for childhood cancer. *J Natl Cancer Inst*. 1987;78(3):459–464.

22. Thirman MJ, Larson RA. Therapy-related myeloid leukemia. *Hematol Oncol Clin N Am.* 1996;10:293–320.

23. Hijiya N, Ness KK, Ribeiro RC, Hudson MM. Acute leukemia as a secondary malignancy in children and adolescents; current findings and issues. *Cancer.* 2009;115:23–35.

24. Choi DK, Helenowski I, Hijiya N. Secondary malignancies in pediatric cancer survivors: perspectives and review of the literature. *Int J Cancer.* 2014;135:1764–1773.

25. Pui CH, Relling MV. Topoisomerase III inhibitor-related acute myeloid leukemia. *Br J Haematol.* 2000;109(1):13–23.

26. Hijiya N, Hudson MM, Lensing S, et al. Cumulative incidence of secondary neoplasms as a first event after childhood acute lymphoblastic leukemia. *JAMA.* 2007;297:1207–1215.

27. Pederson-Bjergaard J, Philip P. Balanced translocations involving chromosome bands 11q23 and 21q22 are highly characteristic of myelodysplasia and leukemia following therapy with cytostatic agents targeting at DNA-topoisomerase II. *Blood.* 1991;78:1147–1148.

28. Kamiya K, Ozasa K, Akiba S, et al. From Hiroshima and Nagasaki to Fukushima 1: long-term effects of radiation exposure on health. *Lancet.* 2015;386:469–478.

29. Friedman DL, Whitton J, Leisenring W, et al. Subsequent neoplasms in 5-year survivors of childhood cancer: the Childhood Cancer Survivor Study. *J Natl Cancer Inst.* 2010;102:1083–1095.

30. Schauer DA, Linton OW. NCRP report no. 160. Ionizing radiation exposure of the population of the United States, medical exposure – are we doing less with more and is there a role for health physicists? *Health Phys.* 2009;97:1–5.

31. Pearce MS, Salotti JA, Little MP, et al. Radiation exposure from CT scans in childhood and subsequent risk of leukaemia and brain tumours: a retrospective cohort study. *Lancet.* 2012;380:499–505.

32. Matthews JD, Forsythe AV, Brady Z, et al. Cancer risk in 680,000 people exposed to computed tomography scans in childhood or adolescence: data linkage study of 11 million Australians. *BMJ.* 2013;346:123–160.

33. Migloretti DL, Johnson E, Williams A, et al. The use of computed tomography in pediatrics and the associated radiation exposure and estimated cancer risk. *JAMA Pediatr.* 2013;167(8):701–707.

34. Goh YI, Bollano E, Einsarson TR, Koren G. Prenatal multivitamine supplementation and rates of pediatric cancers: a meta-analysis. *Clin Pharmacol Ther.* 2007;81(5):685–691.

35. Wigle DT, Turner MC, Krewski D. A systematic review and meta-analysis of childhood leukemia and parental occupational pesticide exposure. *Environ Health Perspect.* 2009;117(10):1505–1513.

36. Chen M, Chang C, Tao L, Lu C. Residential exposure to pesticides during childhood and childhood cancers: a meta-analysis. *Pediatrics.* 2015;136(4):719–729.

37. Klimentopoulou A, Antonopoulos CN, Papadopoulou C, et al. Maternal smoking during pregnancy and risk for childhood leukemia: a nationwide case-control study in Greece and meta-analysis. *Pediatr Blood Cancer.* 2012;58(3):344–351.

38. Latino-Martel P, Chan DS, Druesne-Pecollo N, Barrandon E, Hercberg S, Norat T. Maternal alcohol consumption during pregnancy and risk of childhood leukemia: systematic review and meta-analysis. *Cancer Epidemiol Biomarkers Prev.* 2010;19(5):1238–1260.

39. Urayama KY, Buffler PA, Gallagher ER, Ayoob JM, Ma X. A meta-analysis of the association between daycare attendance and childhood acute lymphoblastic leukemia. *Am J Epidemiol.* 2012;175(1):43–53.

40. Zhao L, Liu X, Wang C, et al. Magnetic fields exposure and childhood leukemia risk: a meta-analysis based on 11,699 cases and 13,194 controls. *Leuk Res.* 2014;38(3):269–274.

41. Shuz J, Weihkopf T, Kaatsch P. Medication use during pregnancy and the risk of childhood cancer in the offspring. *Eur J Pediatr.* 2007;166:433–441.

42. Stalberg K, Haglund B, Stromberg B, Kieler H. Prenatal exposure to medicines and the risk of childhood brain tumor. *Cancer Epidemiol.* 2010;34:400–404.

43. Vinson F, Merhi M, Baldi I, Raynal H, Garnet-Payrastre L. Exposure to pesticides and risk f childhood cancer; a meta-analysis of recent epidemiological studies. *Occup Environ Med.* 2011;68:694–702.

44. Van Maele-Fabry G, Hoet P, Lison D. Parental occupational exposure to pesticides as risk factor for brain tumors in children and young adults; a systematic review and meta-analysis. *Environ Int.* 2013;56:19–31.

45. Huncharek M, Kupelnick B, Lkassen H. Maternal smoking during pregnancy and the risk of childhood brain tumors: a meta-analysis of 6566 subjects from twelve epidemiological studies. *J Neurooncol.* 2002;57:51–57.

46. Milne E, Greenop KR, Scott RJ, et al. Parental alcohol consumption and risk of childhood acute lymphoblastic leukemia and brain tumors. *Cancer Causes Control.* 2013;24:391–402.

47. Harding NJ, Birch JM, Hepworth SJ, McKinney PA. Infectious exposures in the first year of life and risk of central nervous system tumors in children: analysis of day care, social contact and overcrowding. *Cancer Causes Control.* 2009;20:129–136.

48. Shaw AK, Li P, Infante-Rivard C. Early infection and risk of childhood brain tumors (Canada). *Cancer Causes Control.* 2006;17:1267–1274.

49. Harding NJ, Birch JM, Hepsworth SJ, McKinney PA. Breastfeeding and risk of childhood CNS tumors. *Br J Cancer.* 2007;96:815–817.

50. Ha M, Im H, Lee M, et al. Radio-frequency radiation exposure from AM radio transmitters and childhood leukemia and brain cancer. *Am J Epidemiol.* 2007;166:270–279.

51. Mezei G, Gadallah M, Kheifets L. Residential magnetic field exposure and childhood brain cancer: a meta-analysis. *Epidemiology.* 2008;19:424–430.

52. Aydin D, Feychting M, Schuz J, et al. Mobile phone se and brain tumors in children and adolescents: a multicenter case-control study. *J Natl Cancer Inst.* 2011;103:1264–1275.

53. O'Neill KA, Murphy MF, Bunch KJ, et al. Infant birthweight and risks of childhood cancer: international population-based case control studies of 40,000 cases. *Int J Epidemiol.* 2015;44(1):153–168.

54. Hjalgrim LL, Westergaard T, Rostgaard K, et al. Birth weight as a risk factor for childhood leukemia: a meta-analysis of 18 epidemiologic studies. *Am J Epidemiol.* 2003;158(8):724–735.

55. Harder T, Plagemann A, Harder A. Birth weight and subsequent risk of childhood primary brain tumors: a meta-analysis. *Am J Epidemiol.* 2008;168(4):366–373.

56. Harder T, Plagemann A, Harder A. Birth weight and risks of neuroblastoma: a meta-analysis. *Int J Epidemiol.* 2010;39(3):746–756.

57. Chu A, Heck JE, Ribeiro KB, et al. Wilms' tumour: a systematic review of risk factors and meta-analysis. *Paediatr Perinat Epidemiol.* 2010;24(5):449–469.

58. Milne E, Greenop KR, Metayer C, et al. Fetal growth and childhood acute lymphoblastic leukemia: findings from the childhood leukemia international consortium. *Int J Cancer.* 2013;133(12):2968–2979.

59. Caughey RW, Michels KB. Birth weight and childhood leukemia: a meta-analysis and review of the current evidence. *Int J Cancer.* 2009;124(11):2658–2670.

60. Spector LG, Pauumala SE, Carozza S, et al. Cancer risk among children with very low birth weights. *Pediatrics.* 2009;124(1):96–104.

61. Ross JA, Perentesis JP, Robison LL, Davies SM. Big babies and infant leukemia: a role for insulin-like growth factor-1? *Cancer Causes Control.* 1996;7(5):553–559.

62. Turcotte LM, Georgieff MK, Ross JA, et al. Neonatal medical exposures and characteristics of low birth weight hepatoblastoma cases: a report from the Children's Oncology Group. *Pediatr Blood Cancer.* 2014;16(11).

63. Yip BH, Pawitan Y, Czene K. Parental age and risk of childhood cancers: a population-based cohort study from Sweden. *Int J Epidemiol.* 2006;35:1495–1503.

64. Dockerty JD, Draper G, Vincent T, Rowan SD, Bunch KJ. Case controls study of parental age, parity, and socioeconomic level in relation to childhood cancer. *Int J Epidemiol.* 2001;30:1428–1437.

65. Johnson KJ, Carozza S, Chow EJ, et al. Parental age and risk of childhood cancer: a pooled analysis. *Epidemiology.* 2009;20(4):475–483.

66. Narod SA, Stiller C, Lenoir GM. An estimate of the heritable fraction of childhood cancer. *Br J Cancer.* 1991;63:993–999.

67. Zhang J, Walsh MF, Wu G, et al. Germline mutations in predisposition genes in pediatric cancer. *New Engl J Med.* 2015;373:2336–2346.

68. Vogelstein B, Kinzler KW. Cancer genes and the pathways they control. *Nat Med.* 2004;10:789–799.

# CHAPTER 2

# The Genetic Evaluation of a Child With Cancer

NATHANIEL H. ROBIN, MD • ANNA C.E. HURST, MD, MS

## INTRODUCTION

A child with cancer presents a special and difficult challenge to both the healthcare team and the child's family. Parents are understandably overwhelmed with all of the medical concerns that the diagnosis of cancer brings. "What are the treatments?" "Will they work?" "Will my child survive?" These questions about the child's care, along with all the associated complex emotions, are further complicated by the array of healthcare providers—doctors, nurses, pharmacists, and social workers who will be involved in the child's care.

Although concerns are correctly focused on treating the child's cancer, another question that arises at some point is, "What caused the cancer?" For most instances of pediatric cancer, the answer is unknown. As is discussed in Chapter 4, cancer typically arises as a consequence of a collection of genetic mutations that are random events and under no known control. However, for a subset of cases, cancer is a manifestation of an underlying genetic syndrome. It is crucial to recognize a genetic syndrome, as the diagnosis may have significant ramifications for the treatment of the child's cancer, the future health of the child, and risks to family members.

Although genetic syndromes are rare conditions, taken as a group they are common enough that a pediatric oncologist will likely follow several children with genetic diagnoses, perhaps even unrecognized. With an overwhelming number of individual genetic syndromes, it is understandably not expected of the oncologist physician to be knowledgeable of each of the variable phenotypic presentations, especially when he/she is faced with the many other, more immediate concerns regarding the child's medical care.

The purpose of this chapter is to eliminate the mystery behind the clinical genetics evaluation, reviewing the clinical geneticist's role and illustrating how a clinical genetics evaluation can provide valuable information for the parents and other family members as well as to the healthcare team, while helping the oncologist identify appropriate referrals. We discuss how the geneticist evaluates a patient to identify these additional findings that would point to an underlying genetic cause of a child's cancer. Chapters 6 and 7 will delve into more detail about specific cancer syndromes, how they manifest, and the important clues to diagnosing them.

## THE BENEFITS OF MAKING A GENETIC DIAGNOSIS

A genetics evaluation can be quite complex, involving detailed medical and family histories, a specialized physical examination, and genetic testing. The goal, however, is clear—to determine if the patient's presenting finding is isolated or represents one component of an underlying genetic syndrome, and if so, which one. One common and unfortunate misconception is that such a determination is pointless if the condition cannot be "fixed."

Although the underlying genetic variation itself cannot be changed, for an increasing number of genetically determined conditions, accurate identification of the genetic cause may alter management. This is especially true for pediatric cancer, as a genetic diagnosis may alter the child's overall care. Additionally, making a genetic diagnosis will permit accurate prognostication and recurrence risk counseling, inform long-term surveillance and management decisions, and assist in the identification of appropriate social support resources. These are summarized in Box 2.1.

To illustrate the significance of making a genetic diagnosis, let us consider a 4-year-old boy with an osteosarcoma. Although the vast majority of osteosarcomas are isolated, a small percent occurs as part of Li-Fraumeni syndrome, caused by mutations in the *TP53* gene. This may be recognized by identifying other affected individuals with cancers in the family or by the earlier than typical presentation for the child's osteosarcoma.

> **BOX 2.1**
> **Benefits of a Diagnosis**
>
> Establishing and identifying an underlying genetic diagnosis can be of great utility to the child and family affected by pediatric cancer.
> - Improve direct healthcare management
> - Establish accurate risks for secondary malignancies
> - Improve and personalize prognosis
> - Identify the risk to family members to also be affected
> - Initiate screening protocols for at-risk family members
> - Provide recurrence risk information

> **BOX 2.2**
> **Pediatric Oncology-Related Indications for Referral to a Geneticist**
>
> - Child with a rare childhood cancer
> - Child with a childhood cancer with strong genetic component (i.e., retinoblastoma, hemangioblastoma)
> - Child with cancer and other medical issues (e.g., birth defects, unusual facial appearance, intellectual disability, undergrowth/overgrowth)
> - Family history of multiple individuals with cancer, especially early onset or related cancers
> - Parent or first-degree relative with a known cancer syndrome or identified cancer gene mutation

If the child's osteosarcoma was isolated, treatment options would include radiation, something that should be avoided when possible if the child has Li-Fraumeni syndrome. He would also need to have surveillance for other tumors. His first-degree family members should be tested for the *TP53* mutation, as affected family members would also be offered enrollment in a tumor surveillance protocol. Lastly, the patient and all affected family members would be advised that they have a 50% risk of passing on the mutation in each pregnancy. For some that number may seem low, as they expected all of their offspring to inherit the "family curse." Of course, at-risk family members who test negative for the *TP53* mutation could know with confidence that they no longer need increased screening, as their cancer risk is not elevated (but remains at general population risk), and their children are not at risk to have the condition. However, this may raise psychosocial concerns similar to survivor's guilt for family members who know they are not at increased cancer risk while others are. Geneticists and genetic counselors are specifically trained to address these issues and how the medical and psychosocial ramifications impact the entire family.

## INDICATIONS FOR A GENETICS REFERRAL

Determining who should be referred for a genetics evaluation can be a difficult question to answer for several reasons. The physician (or parent) may have a perspective on the case that is not the same as a clinical geneticist would. For example, subtle minor facial findings may not be recognized by anyone but a geneticist, or an especially important item in the family history may not be ascertained if the family was not specifically asked about its presence or absence, simply because its importance is not realized.

Understandably, when taking a family history, most clinicians focus on identifying other relatives with tumors, and that is, of course, very important and relevant. But disparate findings, such as sibling with autism or a congenital heart defect, may also provide clues to diagnosing an underlying genetic syndrome. Not surprisingly, the likelihood of a genetic disorder is greater than most nongenetics professionals realize.

Therefore, the "safe" rule for healthcare professionals is that patients should be referred for a clinical genetics evaluation once the clinical genetics evaluation has been considered. That said, there are several clear indications that should prompt a clinical genetics evaluation. Discussed below, these by no means represent a complete list but are examples of the more common and obvious indications (Box 2.2). Some of the more common indications are discussed below.

See Ref. 1 for additional reading.

### The Child With Multiple Anomalies

There are two reasons that a child with a birth defect may develop a cancer. First, the occurrence of the cancer may be a separate, independent event, unrelated to the birth defect. Although this may seem highly unlikely, when examining the probabilities, it becomes clear that this is not uncommon. Birth defects are common. On aggregate, about 1%–3% of all newborns will have a birth defect. Less frequently occurring is pediatric cancer, with an approximate occurrence of 0.35% of children in the United States before the age of 20 years.[2] So the dual occurrence by chance is not as improbable as one might think.

The second possible explanation is that the cancer and birth defect have the same underlying cause—a genetic syndrome. This may be the result of a point mutation in a single gene, a methylation defect of a critical region of expressed genetic material, or a contiguous gene deletion syndrome. Numerous examples of specific cancer syndromes are discussed in Chapters 6 and 7. It should be noted that the presenting feature may vary across the life span.

### The Patient With Developmental Delay

One of the most common reasons for a clinical geneticist to see a patient, particularly a child, is developmental delay. There are many book chapters and review articles that provide a complete discussion of this topic, and several are listed at the end of this chapter. Suffice it to say here that every child with a developmental delay of unknown etiology should be evaluated by a clinical geneticist and have at least "first tier" genetic testing. The current recommendation is a cytogenetic microarray for chromosomal copy number variation as recommended by the American College of Medical Genetics[3] and Genomics and the International Standard Cytogenomic Array Consortium.[4]

It may seem that developmental delay and cancer are entirely unrelated. However, several recent studies have shown that this is not the case. A substantial number of children with abnormalities on tests commonly done to evaluate developmental delay have also been found to have genetic alterations that lead to a predisposition to developing cancer, such as contiguous gene deletions. For example, a deletion of a portion of chromosome 2q37 contains multiple genes and leads to several features, including birth defects, intellectual disability, hypotonia, and cancer predisposition (specifically Wilm's tumors).

The converse is true as well. Many children undergoing treatment for a cancer may exhibit delays in development/learning, which may be attributed to the hospitalizations and treatments for the cancer. Although this may be the reason, a genetic explanation should be considered as well.

### THE GENETICS EVALUATION

The genetics evaluation is very similar in format to a standard medical evaluation. It includes a history and physical examination and is supplemented by laboratory testing. Counseling is provided based on what is found. The genetics evaluation is, however, different in its execution and emphasis. Other chapters describe in detail the genetic counseling process and how genetic testing differs from other medical tests.

For the geneticist, it is the subtle findings, in family history or on physical examination, that are essential in making the diagnosis of a genetic syndrome. Eliciting subtle, unique physical features allows a geneticist to fully evaluate the child's presentation in the context of family history. An accurate syndrome diagnosis can answer the family's questions of, "Why did this happen?" and "What do we do now?" These questions are often not just for themselves but for members of multiple generations within an entire family.

### PERSONAL AND FAMILY HISTORY

The traditional method to identifying a genetic syndrome starts with a detailed medical history, including prenatal and birth history, followed by a physical examination assessing for minor findings. A comprehensive medical history is vital because it is important to know each medical issue, even (especially) those that seem unrelated to the primary problem.

History should begin with the prenatal history, including focusing on fetal growth, ultrasound abnormalities, exposures to medications and substances, and any maternal or fetal complications during the pregnancy or delivery. Birth history including prematurity, neonatal hypoglycemia, and the need for neonatal intensive care could be indicative of conditions such as Beckwith-Wiedemann syndrome. Developmental milestones may be helpful to assess for intellectual disabilities or concerns for conditions such as autism, which may be a feature of *PTEN*-related disorders.

A detailed three to four generation family history may provide information that suggests a genetic disorder. This is especially true when there is a family history of the same condition as that seen in the patient, such as a cancer, even when that cancer was not initially considered as "genetic." Additional findings may become evident with a heightened index of suspicion, such as the occurrence of a second affected family member.

Care should be taken to obtain both maternal and paternal family histories, as each has equal value, even for gender-specific conditions such as ovarian cancer in females in the paternal lineage or prostate cancer in males in the maternal lineage. Furthermore, it should not be assumed that individuals unaffected with cancers are not truly at risk, as variable expression and reduced penetrance are common in hereditary cancer conditions. When inquiring about cancers, ask the specific diagnosis and age of onset. If an individual has more than one oncologic diagnosis, it is helpful to know if the additional diagnoses are metastases or are truly second primary diagnoses. Although some individuals may have trouble recalling some specific information, personal experience has shown that family member's recall can still be extremely useful.

A family history may reveal seemingly incidental information that turns out to be very relevant, such as individuals with birth defects and physical differences, intellectual disability, developmental delays, or recurrent pregnancy loss. For example, for a child with a medulloblastoma, a sibling with cleft lip or palate, or a parent with basal cell skin carcinomas may seem unrelated, but this indicates a diagnosis of nevoid basal cell carcinoma syndrome (formerly called Gorlin syndrome).

However, it is important to remember that not all conditions that occur in multiple family members are due to genetics. Some are caused by nongenetic factors that also cluster in families, such as shared environments. This is true in cancer predisposition syndromes and also other genetic conditions, such as intellectual disability. A classic example is a family with several children with developmental delay/intellectual disability and distinct facial appearance due to repeated maternal alcohol use during pregnancy. Each child likely has fetal alcohol syndrome. Although most physicians and scientists agree that alcohol abuse has clear genetic underpinnings, the children in this example have a common phenotype due to their shared "environmental" influence.

## ISOLATED VERSUS SYNDROMIC

While gathering the many facts of a patient's birth, developmental, and medical history, one attempts to determine if a patient's findings have related themes. Most pediatric cancer instances occur as an isolated finding, without other manifestations or abnormalities. However, for a subset of children, the cancer is one finding in a more complex clinical presentation. In some cases, the other findings have been known for some time. For example, for a child with a newly diagnosed Wilm's tumor, the parents would have long known if there was associated aniridia, hemihyperplasia, or an omphalocele. In such cases, the geneticist's role would to put a name to the underlying syndrome and counsel the parents accordingly if that had not already been done.

In some cases, the geneticist may be the first to identify findings that suggest an underlying cancer syndrome. For example, café-au-lait macules (Fig. 2.1) may have been dismissed as nothing more than "birthmarks." However, they take on more significant meaning in the child with an optic glioma or malignant peripheral nerve sheath tumor because they suggest the diagnosis of neurofibromatosis type 1 (NF1). Although NF1 is a common condition associated with café au lait macules, ruling out a diagnosis of NF1 does not negate the significance of this finding, as children with more rare conditions such as constitutional mismatch repair deficiency syndrome can also display café-au-lait macules. It is important to recognize when one external finding could indicate any one of multiple different genetic syndromes.

There are hundreds of genetic syndromes that are associated with cancer. Some have obvious somatic manifestations, such as Down syndrome or neurofibromatosis type I, whereas others have no obvious physical finding and only carry an increased risk for developing cancer, such as Li-Fraumeni syndrome.

## THE GENETICS PHYSICAL EXAMINATION

The genetics physical examination has several notable differences from the typical medical examination. The genetic examination focuses on identifying the subtle physical findings that represent clues to the underlying genetic syndrome, discussed below. This approach is termed "dysmorphology," which is the study of abnormal form with an emphasis on structural developmental abnormalities. A dysmorphological evaluation of a child (or fetus or adult) looks for unusual physical (or behavioral) characteristics that might provide insight into errors in embryologic or fetal development, major or minor.

A geneticist's thorough physical examination includes measurement of multiple structures and observational assessment for dysmorphic findings. When possible, measurements should be obtained and plotted against standardized growth charts. References such as the *Handbook of Physical Measurements*[5] contain descriptions of the methods by which to obtain precise measurements and accompanying growth charts.

The use of precise terminology is recommended in the description and documentation of the physical examination. Updated preferred terminology can be found in a collection of published articles, "Elements of Morphology: Human Malformation Terminology," https://elementsofmorphology.nih.gov/ which were intended to develop accurate and clear definitions for the terms of the craniofacies, hands, and feet.

For geneticists, the first "vital signs" are growth parameters, including a careful assessment of length, weight, and head circumference. Undergrowth or overgrowth can be not just global, but regional growth differences are also associated with many cancer risks. Macrocephaly is an important marker of many genetic syndromes (such as *PTEN*-related disorders or nevoid basal cell carcinoma syndrome), and microcephaly is

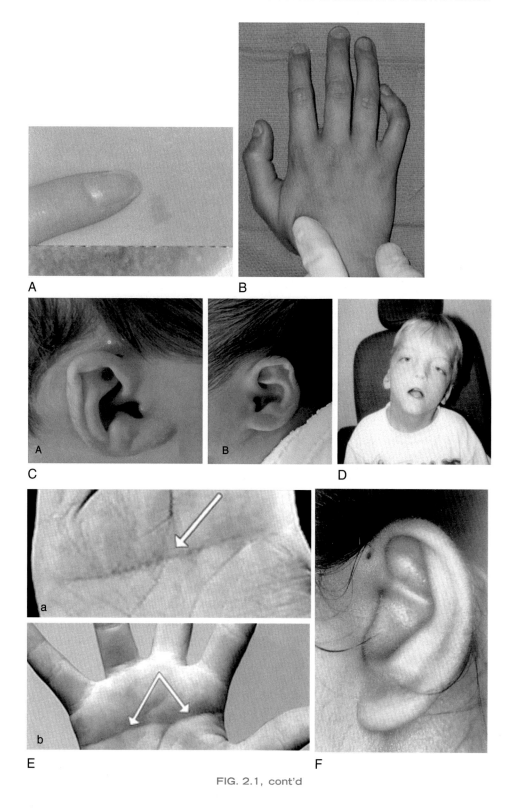

FIG. 2.1, cont'd

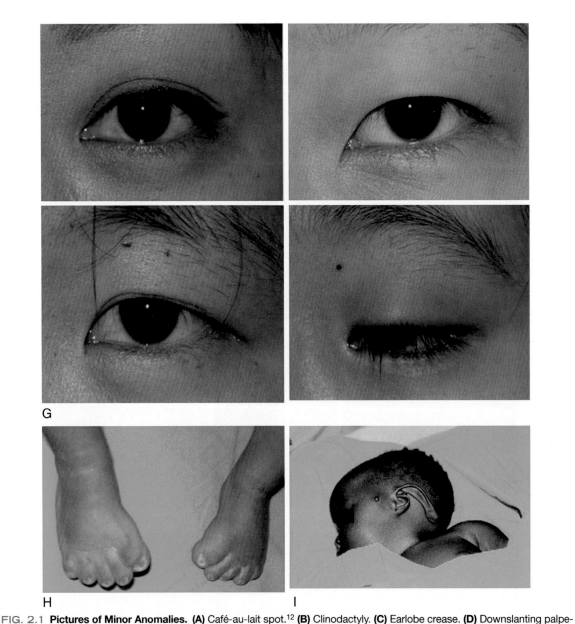

FIG. 2.1 **Pictures of Minor Anomalies.** **(A)** Café-au-lait spot.[12] **(B)** Clinodactyly. **(C)** Earlobe crease. **(D)** Downslanting palpebral fissures. **(E)** Single transverse palmar crease. **(F)** Preauricular pit. **(G)** Epicanthus. **(H)** f 2,3 syndactyly. **(I)** Preauricular tag.
((A) From Kandt RS. Tuberous sclerosis complex and neurofibromatosis type 1: the two most common neurocutaneous diseases. *Neurol Clin*. November 2003;21(4):983–1004. (B) From Goldfarb CA, Wall LB. Osteotomy for clinodactyly. *J Hand Surg Am*. June 2015;40(6):1220–1224. http://dx.doi.org/10.1016/j.jhsa.2015.03.003. Epub 2015 Apr 16. (C) From Jedlińska D, Kowalska-Czech J, Wójcicka-Kowalczyk C, et al. The variety of clinical and diagnostic difficulties and Beckwith Wiedemann syndrome in the neonatal period diversity of Beckwith-Wiedemann syndrome and complexity of molecular diagnosis during neonatal period. *Pediatrics*. July–August 2016;91(4):350–358. (D) From Lee WB, O'Halloran HS, Grossfeld PD, et al. Ocular findings in Jacobsen syndrome. *J AAPOS*. April 2004;8(2):141–145. (E) From Zvi Shamir E, Levy A, Morris CS, et al. Do biometric parameters of the hand differentiate schizophrenia from other psychiatric disorders? A comparative evaluation using three mental health modules. *Psychiatry Res*. August 30, 2015;228(3):425–430. http://dx.doi.org/10.1016/j.psychres.2015.06.020. Epub 2015 Jun 27. (F) From Prabhu NT, Alexander S, John R. Branchio-oto-renal syndrome with generalized microdontia: case report. *Oral Surg Oral Med Oral Pathol Oral Radiol Endod*. February 1999;87(2):180–183. (G) From Lai CS, Lai CH, Wu YC, Chang KP, Lee SS, Lin SD. Medial epicanthoplasty based on anatomic variations. *J Plast Reconstr Aesthet Surg*. September 2012;65(9):1182–1187. http://dx.doi.org/10.1016/j.bjps.2011.12.038. Epub 2012 Jun 30. (H) From Shawky RM, Elkhalek HSA, Al-Fahham MM, et al. Oral-facial-digital syndrome with mesoaxial polysyndactyly, common AV canal, hirschsprung disease and sacral dysgenesis: probably a transitional type between II, VI, variant of type VI or a new type. *Egypt J Med Hum Genet*. 2014;15(3):305–310. (I) From James JH. Congenital cleft ear: a case report. *Br J Plast Surg*. December 2004;57(8):792–793.)

seen in many chromosomal deletion syndromes that can affect regions containing cancer predisposition genes.

The evaluation should include full skin examination assessing for congenital or acquired hyperpigmentation or hypopigmentation, growths (such as lipomas), and telangiectasias. The distribution of pigmentary changes should be closely examined, as streaking hyperpigmentation is a sign of tissue mosaicism, indicating genetic differences that may not be identified on routine blood testing. The hair, nails, and teeth should also be closely examined as part of the examination, and/or families should be asked about growth patterns or any irregularities that they have noted. For example, several dark spots around the mouth may not seem to be important in a teenager with newly diagnosed colon cancer, but they suggest the diagnosis of Peutz-Jeghers syndrome.

The remaining examination is best proceeded from head to toe, including the face and orbits, ears, nose, mouth, and jaw. Eye examination should include periorbital features (spacing of eyes, palpebral fissure size, and slanting) and ocular structures (pupils and fundus, if able). Care should be taken to assess for symmetry and the gestalt appearance of how each region "fits" in the overall appearance of the face. Measurements can be extremely useful in determining if a structure is objectively big or small. A common adage among clinical geneticists is "don't say it's big or small without measuring it first," as a structure may appear small or large but merely be out of proportion to other structures.

Chest and abdominal examinations should include auscultation, as some congenital heart defects may not have been noted prior. (The cardiac auscultation is also a time when young patients in the room become quiet and still, and the careful examiner can use this time to silently observe the face in close detail.)

Genitourinary examinations can also reveal signs of hypogonadism or even dermatologic changes such as freckling of the glans penis as seen in *PTEN*-related disorders.

The extremities and musculoskeletal system exam can reveal obvious anomalies, such as absent or triphalangeal thumbs, or more subtle findings, such as broad digits, clinodactyly, or asymmetric palmar creases. Limb asymmetry may be hemihyperplasia, which could indicate a systemic syndrome or tissue mosaicism.

A full neurologic examination is also an important tool to assess for subtle deficits, although it is important to know the child's prior baseline and what deficits may have been acquired during any cancer management or treatment (such as postsurgical changes).

## THE SIGNIFICANCE OF MINOR ANOMALIES

*The best clues are the rarest. Quite often, these are not the most obvious anomalies nor even the ones that have the greatest significance for the patient's health.*

JON AASE, MD

The physical examination may reveal "minor anomalies," which may be another common indication for referral to the geneticist. Minor anomalies are physical variations that may be seen in the general population but may also provide subtle clues to a genetic diagnosis (Fig. 2.2; Table 2.1). These may be related to the facial features and result in the patient having an unusual facial appearance. Such patients are referred to as "dysmorphic," reflecting the fact that their facial appearance is atypical, especially when compared with family members. Many years ago such patients were often referred to as "FLKs" or "funny looking kids," but such terms are strongly discouraged today, although they are unfortunately still used by some healthcare professionals who have limited experience with patients with special needs.

By definition, minor anomalies have little to no medical significance, but as indicated in Dr. Aase's quote, it is by identifying minor anomalies that most genetic syndromes are diagnosed. Approximately one in seven babies have one minor anomaly; however, multiple minor anomalies raise the chance that there is a major anomaly also present,[6-8] which also leads to the possibility of a genetic syndrome.

Determination of an "atypical" facial appearance is based on both an individual observer's subjective assessment and objective measures. Some aspects can be measured, such as eye spacing and ear length, and compared with accepted normal values. Other findings, such as lip contour and ear shape, are based on the viewer's experience and are therefore somewhat subjective. Some commonly described minor anomalies are seen in Fig. 2.1.

It is important to remember that minor anomalies are important only in the context within which they are viewed. For example, single transverse palmar creases occur in up to 4% of the general population. If seen in an otherwise healthy individual, they have little importance. However, when seen in a hypotonic newborn with a flattened midface, upslanting palpebral fissures, and an atrial-ventricular canal cardiac defect, the diagnosis of Down syndrome should be strongly considered.

These subtle "minor" abnormal findings are typically only of cosmetic significance, distinguishing them from more severe congenital anomalies, which are termed "major anomalies." Major anomalies include birth defects, but also other differences that have functional significance and may require surgical or medical management, such as extreme undergrowth or overgrowth or profound intellectual disabilities.

## HOW TO IDENTIFY A GENETIC SYNDROME/ MAKE A DIAGNOSIS

How does a clinical geneticist sort through the information obtained through the medical and family histories and physical examination to reach a genetic syndrome diagnosis?

Most physicians are familiar with making diagnoses when clear familial patterns are present (such as in familial retinoblastoma), when a specific tumor type is associated with certain syndromes (Wilm's tumor), or when a known syndrome is present and focused tumor screening is needed (Beckwith-Wiedemann syndrome). The geneticist is most useful when a systems-based approach is needed to evaluate for minor and major anomalies and to put these findings in the context of the medical and family history.[9]

In some instances, a geneticist will immediately recognize the facial characteristics as those of a specific genetic syndrome on seeing a child. The geneticist will

This guide is not intended to be all-inclusive, but may serve as a framework by which to approach the findings of significance in an examination for dysmorphic findings and possible genetic conditions.

**Growth/Body Parameters**

| Height | _____ cm | _____ % |
|---|---|---|
| Weight | _____ kg | _____ % |
| Occipitofrontal circumference (OFC) | _____ cm | _____ % |
| Upper segment: Lower segment ratio _____ | | |

**Craniofacial**–assess for an overall gestalt, but also examine features individually. Take note of overt birth defects (oral clefting, ocular colobomas) but also minor descriptions and any asymmetry. May also be helpful to note if parents or other family members share these findings.

| | Description/Noted Findings |
|---|---|
| Cranium–shape | |
| Fontanelle–size, if open | |
| Hair – position and number of whorls, texture, hairline | |
| Face–overall appearance | (Ex: long, flat, broad, coarse, narrow, round, triangular) |
| Periorbital–spacing, palpebral fissures, ocular abnormalities | Outer canthus   _____ cm _____ %<br>Inner canthus   _____ cm _____ %<br>Inner pupillary   _____ cm _____ % |
| Malar region | |
| Ears–structure, size, placement, rotation, landmarks, pits/tags | Ear length   _____ cm _____ % |
| Nose–nasal bridge, tip, alae | |
| Perioral–philtrum, lip | |
| Oral–size and shape of mouth, uvula | |
| Dental–tooth presence, spacing, appearance | |
| Mandibular | (Ex: prognathism, micrognathia, retrognathia) |

**FIG. 2.2 Physical Exam Findings of Significance in the Pediatric Oncologic Genetic Exam.** (Adapted from Gripp (2013) and Miles (2008).

**Skeletal Findings**

| | |
|---|---|
| Limbs – shortening, asymmetry, hemihyperplasia | |
| Hands–placement and deviation of hands and fingers, clinodactyly, persistence of fetal fingertip pads, dermatoglyphic patterns, nail development | Hand length _____ cm _____% <br> Middle finger length _____ cm _____% |
| Feet– poly/syndactyly, broad toes, nail development | Foot length _____ cm _____% |
| Joints– assess for hypermobility, contractures | |

**Genitalia**

| | |
|---|---|
| Tanner Stage– delayed/precocious puberty | Tanner Stage _____ |
| Males: penile length, testicular volume, hypospadias, scrotal development | |
| Anal placement | |

**Skin**

| | |
|---|---|
| Pigmentation–streaking, birthmarks, hyper/hypopigmented lesions | |
| Vasculature–capillary naevus, telangeiectasias, bruising | |

*Adapted from Gripp, 2013 and Miles, 2008.*

FIG. 2.2, cont'd

---

**TABLE 2.1**
**Major Versus Minor Anomalies**

| Major | Minor |
|---|---|
| Physical differences with a significant functional, medical, or cosmetic implication. Reflects abnormal development and may require surgical interventions to restore normal function | Physical variation with little or no medical or cosmetic effect. Although minor anomalies rarely require surgical or medical intervention, they may provide important clues to the diagnostician |
| Examples: <br> • Cleft lip and palate <br> • Severe micrognathia <br> • Macroglossia <br> • Congenital heart defects <br> • Neural tube defects (anencephaly, spina bifida) <br> • Omphalocele/gastroschisis <br> • Limb deficiencies | Examples: <br> • Abnormal hair whorls <br> • Epicanthal folds <br> • Preauricular pits or tags <br> • Clinodactyly (incurving of the finger) <br> • Supernummary nipples <br> • Single transverse palmar crease <br> • Umbilical hernia <br> • Sacral dimple |

---

**BOX 2.3**
Practical Genetic Resources for the Clinician

**THESE RESOURCES CAN ASSIST IN MAKING A DIAGNOSIS**

- OMIM—omim.org

  Online catalog of human genes and genetic disorders. Can search by clinical feature, gene, or condition name. Useful tools are the "clinical synopsis" and clinical resources link to external sites.

- Phenomizer—compbio.charite.de/phenomizer

  A drag-and-drop method of using Human Phenotype Ontology (diagnostic terms) to create a differential diagnosis ranked by *p*-values.

- Face2Gene—App and website—fdna.com

  Import photograph into this HIPAA-compliant tool to create a differential diagnosis using facial recognition software. View a "gestalt" match or enter features for more specificity. Features an "unknowns forum" for clinicians and "academy" of dysmorphology-based quizzes.

- GeneTests—genetests.org

  Directory of clinical laboratory test listings and clinic locations. Can search by condition or gene name to find where testing can be performed; links to those sites.

**THESE RESOURCES PROVIDE INFORMATION ABOUT SPECIFIC GENETIC SYNDROMES**

- GeneReviews—genereviews.org

  A point-of-care resource for busy clinicians, peer-reviewed, written by field experts. Contains relevant, medically actionable information on over 670 conditions.

- Unique—rarechromo.org

  A collection of informative "Disorder Guides" for a variety of chromosome and single-gene conditions. Offers support for families and siblings. Has a guide about what to expect at a clinical genetics appointment.

- Genetics Home Reference—ghr.nlm.nih.gov

  Consumer-friendly information about human genetics from the US National Library of Medicine. Search by specific conditions or general genetics topics.

- Condition-Specific Guidelines—go to geneticsinprimarycare.aap.org→Genetics in Your Practice→Patient Management and Guidelines

  Centralized location for collection of published guidelines and landmark papers for 17 of the most common genetic conditions.

**THESE RESOURCES PROVIDE EDUCATIONAL MATERIAL ABOUT AND MANAGEMENT GUIDELINES FOR SPECIFIC GENETIC CONDITIONS**

- Genetics in Primary Care—geneticsinprimarycare.aap.org

  Information and tools for incorporating genetics into daily practice. Provides toolkits, webinars, and educational content on topics such as medical homes, transitioning care, quality improvement, and ethical issues in genetics.

---

see the child's dysmorphic findings not individually but as a unit and identifies the specific syndrome by an overall gestalt. For example, a child with an omphalocele who has a large tongue and a midline hemangioma between his/her eyebrows would make the experienced clinician immediately consider Beckwith-Wiedemann syndrome.

Such a "snap" diagnosis relies on the clinician's experience and memory, and although it does occur, it is unfortunately not common. Even the most experienced geneticist is typically left to use various resources (books and electronic databases) in an effort to make a diagnosis. These are listed in Box 2.3. It should be noted that, while there are many excellent online resources, there are many books that remain valuable when trying to identify a genetic syndrome. Two commonly used are *Smith's Recognizable Patterns of Human Malformation*[10] and *Gorlin's Syndromes of the Head and Neck.*[11] Even with the modern electronic databases listed in Box 2.3, these books continue to be very valuable and easy-to-use resources when trying to find what syndromes are associated with a specific finding.

## REEVALUATION AND FOLLOW-UP

In some cases, an older child or young adult may have been evaluated when they were younger, and no diagnosis was made. In that case a reevaluation is certainly worthwhile. Each year, new genetics syndromes are identified based on newly emerging clinical findings or because of advances in genetic testing. Even the oldest genetic test—cytogenetic analysis—has improved in quality substantially in the past decade. For these reasons, any child who does not have a diagnosis should be reevaluated periodically, typically every 2–3 years. This general principle applies to any patient whom a clinical geneticist sees, regardless of the indication. In some cases, the interval should be even shorter, as it is unpredictable when a new appropriate test will become available.

## REFERENCES

1. Hampel H, Bennett RL, Buchanan A, Pearlman R, Wiesner GL. A practice guideline from the American College of Medical Genetics and Genomics and the National Society of Genetic Counselors: referral indications for cancer predisposition assessment. *Genet Med.* 2015;17(1):70–87.
2. Howlader N, Noone AM, Krapcho M, et al., eds. *SEER Cancer Statistics Review, 1975-2013.* Bethesda, MD: National Cancer Institute; April 2016. http://seer.cancer.gov/csr/1975_2013/. Based on November 2015 SEER data submission, posted to the SEER web site.
3. Manning M, Hudgins L. Array-based technology and recommendations for utilization in medical genetics practice for detection of chromosomal abnormalities. *Genet Med.* 2010;12(11):742–745.
4. Miller DT, Adam MP, Aradhya S, et al. Consensus statement: chromosomal microarray is a first-tier clinical diagnostic test for individuals with developmental disabilities or congenital anomalies. *Am J Hum Genet.* 2010;86(5):749–764.
5. Gripp KW, Slavotinek AM, Hall JG, Allanson JE. *Handbook of Normal Physical Measurements.* 3rd ed. Oxford University Press; 2013.
6. Leppig KA, Werler MM, Cann CI, Cook CA, Holmes LB. Predictive value of minor anomalies. Association with major malformations. *J Pediatr.* 1987;110:531–537.
7. Marden PM, Smith DW, McDonald MJ. Congenital anomalies in the newborn infant, including minor variations. A study of 4,412 babies by surface examination for anomalies and buccal smear for sex chromatin. *J Pediatr.* 1964;64:357–371.
8. Mehes K, Mestyan J, Knoch V, Vinceller M. Minor malformation in the neonate. *Helv Pediatr Acta.* 1973;28:477–483.
9. Clericuzio C. Recognition and management of childhood cancer syndromes: a systems approach. *Am J Med Genet.* 1999;89:81–90.
10. Jones KL, Jones M, del Campo M. *Smith's Recognizable Patterns of Human Malformation.* 7th ed. Philadelphia: Elsevier Saunders; 2013.
11. Hennekam RCM, Krantz ID, Allanson JE. *Gorlin's Syndromes of the Head and Neck.* 5th ed. Oxford, UK: Oxford publishing; 2010.
12. Nebesio TD, Eugester EA. Café Au Lait macules and axillary freckling. *Curr Probl Pediatr Adolesc Health Care.* 2007;37:50–72.
13. Miles JH, Takahashi TN, Hong J, et al. Development and validation of a measure of dysmorphology: useful for autism subgroup classification. *Am J Med Genet A.* 2008;146A(9):1101–1116.

## FURTHER READING

1. Aase J. *Diagnostic Dysmorphology.* New York: Plenum Medical Book Co; 1990.
2. Jongmans MCJ, Loeffen JLCM, Waanders E, et al. Recognition of genetic predisposition in pediatric cancer patients: an easy-to-use selection tool. *Eur J Med Genet.* 2016;59(3):116–125.
3. Robin NH. It does matter: the importance of making the diagnosis of a genetic syndrome. *Curr Opin Pediatr.* 2006;18(6):595–597.
4. Bankier A, Keith CG. Possum: a microcomputer laser videodisk syndrome information system. *Ophthalmic Paediatr Genet.* 1989;10:51–52.
5. Winter RM, Baratitser M. *The London Dysmorphology Database: A Computerized Database for the Diagnosis of Rare Dysmorphic Syndromes.* 5th ed. Oxford university Press; 1998.

# CHAPTER 3

# Genetic Counseling

SONJA HIGGINS, MS, CGC

## INTRODUCTION TO GENETIC COUNSELING

In this chapter, we aim to familiarize practitioners with genetic counseling. Genetic counselors help guide families through the process of determining whether cancer(s) in a family is due to a hereditary cause, how this information may affect treatment and surveillance, and what impact such a diagnosis may have on family members.[1] Although the general process is similar regardless of the type of patient (child or adult) or indication (congenital anomaly, pregnancy), the approach to the patient with, or at risk for, cancer has unique features. That being said, it is important to understand genetic counseling, in general, as a basis to understand cancer genetic counseling.

A scope of practice document created by members of the National Society of Genetic Counselors (NSGC), in part, defines genetic counselors as "health professionals with specialized education, training and experience in medical genetics and counseling who help people understand and adapt to the implications of genetic contributions to disease."[2] A definition of genetic counseling created by NSGC members in 2006 states:

> Genetic counseling is the process of helping people understand and adapt to the medical, psychological and familial implications of genetic contributions to disease. This process integrates the following:
> Interpretation of family and medical histories to assess the chance of disease occurrence or recurrence.
> Education about inheritance, testing management, prevention, resources and research.
> Counseling to promote informed choices and adaptation to the risk or condition.[3]

Genetic counselors hold master's degrees in genetic counseling from graduate programs accredited by the American Board of Genetic Counseling. The first class of genetic counselors graduated in 1971, and there are currently 36 accredited genetic counseling programs in the United States. There are ~4000 genetic counselors nationwide.[4] Many of the first genetic counselors practiced in the areas of prenatal or pediatric counseling. However, as more knowledge about hereditary cancer predisposition was gained, there was growth in the number of genetic counselors practicing in cancer

settings. By 2002, there were more genetic counselors practicing in cancer than in pediatrics. Currently, the NSGC reports that more genetic counselors practice in cancer than in either prenatal or pediatric settings, making cancer the most common subspecialty in genetic counseling.[5]

The increased demand for cancer genetic counselors comes in part from recommendations by organizations such as the American Society of Clinical Oncology, which issued a statement recommending clinical oncologists to assess whether patients with cancer have an inherited form of cancer.[6] Still, there are far fewer cancer genetic counselors than oncology practices. Many cancer centers do not have a genetic counselor available on site. Because of this, referrals are often made to major medical centers. When patients are not able to travel to larger centers for these more specialized services, there are sometimes options to receive the services through telemedicine. In other cases, the local oncology office provides the service through a nurse with specialized training in cancer genetics. The American Society of Oncology published a policy statement update in 2015 that affirmed the need for those providing care to cancer patients to have sufficient education and training in the genetics of cancer.[7]

The hallmark of genetic counseling is that there is an emphasis on the communication process that occurs between the genetic counselor and the patient and his/her family.[3] Genetic counseling is not simply a teaching session, although teaching is an important element. The genetic counselor strives to gather and provide information in an easily understandable manner while giving attention to the emotional impact of the conversation. In many settings, a genetic counselor typically works with a medical geneticist, a physician with specialized training in genetics. The genetic counselor gathers information and provides a summary of the case to the medical geneticist before his/her evaluation. The genetic counselor also spends time with the family after the medical geneticist has completed his/her assessment to continue the education and support roles. However, in a cancer setting, the genetic counselor may collaborate with an oncologist or a surgeon rather than a medical geneticist and is the expert rounding out the team of care for the family. Unlike in pediatric, prenatal, or general adult genetics settings, a genetic counselor in a cancer genetics setting may work more autonomously, meaning he/she is not under the direct supervision of a geneticist, oncologist, or surgeon. This is largely because a physical examination may not be necessary in the evaluation of some cancer genetic counseling patients.

Another distinguishing element of genetic counseling is attention to patient autonomy because the patients navigate their healthcare decisions. Usually, the genetic counselor provides a discussion of the pros and cons of testing and/or management options in a nondirective manner and helps the family decide how they would like to proceed. This model of care is particularly suited to prenatal situations, which were most common early in the history of genetic counseling. However, in the case of pediatric cancer genetic counseling, genetic test results may impact cancer treatment and long-term management. These medical management recommendations may have significant benefits for the patient and for family members who are diagnosed with the same cancer predisposition syndrome. Providing recommendations regarding care is a change from the original practice of nondirectiveness in genetic counseling. In cases of cancer, genetic counselors provide information about how a genetic diagnosis might influence the monitoring and treating of an illness, which requires a more directive approach.[1]

## ELEMENTS OF GENETIC COUNSELING SESSIONS

The best method for understanding the true nature of the encounter with the genetic counselor is to review the steps of the session as they apply to visits with pediatric cancer patients and their families. In the case of pediatric cancer patients, most of the conversation occurs with the parents or the child's caregiver, but depending on the age of the child, it may be appropriate to include the child in some of the conversations as well.

## MEDICAL HISTORY

Taking a careful medical history of the child with cancer is important in providing an assessment of risk for an inherited cancer syndrome. The child has often been through a long course of diagnosis and treatment before the genetic counseling visit. It is important to learn the age of diagnosis, the type of cancer, pathology of the tumor, surgical interventions or other treatments

required, current state of health, plan of surveillance, and any known environmental exposures.[8] The presence of benign tumors or bilateral cancers is important to note. Medical records are important in answering some of these questions. A medical history intake in a pediatric cancer setting will also include general medical and surgical history information as well as developmental history. Parents or caregivers may find it difficult to talk about all the child has endured, particularly if the prognosis is poor or if the child is deceased. Genetic counselors are trained to be compassionate and caring in their questions and responses. They provide short-term psychosocial counseling and may make referrals to other mental health professionals as needed.[1]

## FAMILY HISTORY

One of the most important steps in the genetic counseling process is to take a careful family history with close attention to others in the family with cancer. The presence of several family members with the same or related cancers, especially rare cancers, increases the chance for an inherited cancer syndrome. The family history is drawn as a diagram called a pedigree, with circles and squares representing males and females, respectively, and lines representing relationships connecting them. A three to four generation family history is typically taken unless there are relatives outside of the four generations with cancers. The genetic counselor asks for information about any relative who has had cancer, such as the type of cancer, the age at which it occurred, information regarding the pathology of the cancer (stage and grade, for example), the treatment that was required, and if any genetic testing was ever done or a genetic diagnosis was ever made. If the family history is suggestive of a particular cancer syndrome, then there are often additional specific questions related to the condition that follows. Reviewing all of this information can be an emotionally difficult process when close relatives have struggled and died from cancer. The genetic counselor is attuned to this possibility and stops to acknowledge suffering and loss.[1,8]

In addition to cancer, there are questions about the overall health of other relatives. Characteristic noncancerous conditions/findings can occur in individuals with some cancer syndromes, making it important to ask about the presence of other such features. These may include birth defects, autism, macrocephaly, noncancerous tumors, and other unusual features such as birthmarks. The age and cause of death is documented for first and potentially second degree relatives of the patient. The ancestry of the family is ascertained, given that some cancer syndromes occur with a greater frequency in particular ethnic groups. Because consanguinity increases the chance for cancer syndromes inherited in an autosomal recessive manner, it is important to determine if this is a possibility. Of course, a family history is often biased by patient recall and knowledge. It is best to obtain documentation in the form of medical records when possible, to verify diagnoses of importance to the particular situation.[1,8]

## RISK ASSESSMENT

A careful physical evaluation of a child with cancer by a medical geneticist for noncancerous features of a genetic syndrome can be a benefit when conducting a risk assessment for some syndromes (for more information see Referral Indications for Genetic Counseling section and Chapter 2). Once the medical and family histories of the patient have been obtained and the physical evaluation has been performed (if indicated), an assessment of the level of risk for an inherited cancer syndrome is performed. Most cases of pediatric cancer are not inherited, but risk assessment allows for identification of those that have a higher likelihood to be due to a hereditary cause. Typically, risk for an inherited cancer syndrome can be categorized as high, moderate, or low. Those with a high risk often have several relatives affected with similar types of cancer, early ages of diagnosis, a clear pattern of inheritance in the family (such as autosomal dominant), rare cancers, bilateral cancers, relatives with multiple primary tumors, and the presence of suggestive noncancerous features. In moderate risk scenarios, a family history may have some high-risk features, but not many or all of them, whereas a low-risk family has few of the aforementioned features. A low-risk family would be one in which the cancers present are common and occur at older ages and the affected relatives do not fit any particular pattern of inheritance.[1,8]

When a child is identified as high risk for an inherited cancer syndrome, specific syndromes can be considered for possible diagnosis and testing. Even if a diagnosis is not made, the risk assessment may allow for the recommendation of certain screening interventions (for more information see Result Disclosure section). Being at high risk for an inherited cancer syndrome means that the person may have an increased chance for other cancers and that others in the family are also at risk for cancer.[1,8] Learning this in addition to dealing with a child's cancer diagnosis can cause anxiety for families. Genetic counselors present this risk information as simply as possible to make it easier to

understand in a time of distress. Tools such as visual aids or repetition are used to facilitate understanding. Genetic counselors are also careful to assess understanding of risks discussed so that clarifications can be made if there are misunderstandings.

## DISCUSSION OF GENETIC TESTING

For many genetic conditions, including those with adult onset and/or no medical management implications in childhood, genetic testing is not offered to minors. However, in the realm of pediatric cancer, genetic testing is offered in certain situations. Genetic counselors engage in a thorough discussion of the pros and cons of genetic testing with the parents, and a recommendation is made as to whether genetic testing is appropriate for the child. If the family history and child's medical history or physical evaluations are suggestive of an inherited cancer syndrome, then genetic testing is likely offered. Other factors that are important when considering whether to offer a genetic test or not include whether the test can be clearly interpreted, whether the test results may influence the management or treatment of the child, and whether the child or parent is able to give informed consent as discussed further below. Taking these factors into consideration, a recommendation is made to the family about the appropriateness of a genetic test. If testing is offered, the family ultimately decides whether to proceed.

Genetic counselors strive to ensure that the family understands the type of genetic testing available for the particular condition(s) suspected. Some genetic tests are diagnostic tests, meaning a positive test indicates that the child has a molecular diagnosis of a genetic condition. A screening test indicates whether it is more or less likely that a child has the associated condition. If most diagnostic cancer genetic tests are positive, they indicate a person has a genetic condition and is at increased risk for cancer. Some tests, however, may determine that a person is a carrier for a recessive cancer syndrome, meaning he/she does not have the condition but that a child could be affected.[1,8] Carrier testing is typically not performed in children, given that being identified as a carrier of a genetic condition usually does not impact medical management.

There are a number of factors that can make genetic testing in a cancer setting complicated. For instance, the medical and/or family history may be suspicious for more than one cancer syndrome. Deciding which syndromes and the order in which to test for them requires experience and expertise. Additionally, a particular cancer syndrome may be caused by mutations in more than one gene. It may be necessary to test several genes to rule out or lessen the suspicion for one syndrome. Multigene panel testing may also be justifiable but may include the analysis of genes that are associated with genetic conditions not included in the differential. Some may even be associated with conditions with adult onset that are not typically tested for in childhood. For more information on genetic testing techniques and ethical issues in pediatric cancer genetic testing, see Chapters 5 and 8, respectively. Because of the complexity of genetic testing options, the American Society of Clinical Oncology stated that "providers with particular expertise in cancer risk assessment should be involved in the ordering and interpretation of multigene panels that include genes of uncertain clinical utility and genes not suggested by the patient's personal and/or family history."[7] In some cases there are additional causative genes for a condition that have not yet been identified, and thus if a genetic test for that condition is negative, it does not rule out the condition. The number of causative genes identified in association with each type of cancer is variable. The genetic counselor provides an up-to-date estimation of the likelihood that a genetic test will be informative. Another important consideration for patients is that health insurance does not cover every genetic test, making it more difficult for families to be tested for a number of conditions or genes. Finally, some genetic tests are available on a clinical basis, and others are performed as part of a research study. When a test is available on a clinical basis, the test is performed within a predicted period of time and for a specific cost. When it is part of a research study, there is often no cost, but the testing may take a long time to complete and there may never be a result reported back to the family.[1,8]

## INFORMED CONSENT FOR GENETIC TESTING

Once a family has decided to have genetic testing, the genetic counselor reviews the tests offered in detail to be sure the family has a realistic expectation regarding the result. Box 3.1 lists the elements of a thorough informed consent.

The informed consent process can be lengthy and technical, and there are many potential misconceptions regarding the meaning of genetic test results. Genetic counselors use easy-to-understand language and various teaching strategies to explain the test(s) as well as all of the limitations and implications. They monitor how a family is processing the information and prompt discussion of the family's feeling about the testing.

---

**BOX 3.1**
**Elements of Informed Consent for Genetic Forms of Cancer**

The particular condition suspected and why genetic testing is being offered

The gene or genes being tested and what is known about these genes

How the gene(s) is inherited and risks to family members when a mutation is present

Accuracy of the genetic test—how often the gene being tested is associated with the condition in question and how often the test is uninformative or the result is unclear

When a mutation is present, how the condition may present

The clinical implications of the test result, such as impact on medical care

Logistics, such as turnaround time and cost

The possibility of genetic discrimination with mention of laws such as the Genetic Nondiscrimination Act of 2008

Confidentiality of the result

How the test result can be used to manage and treat the patient

Any other tests that may be available that could provide additional information and/or alternatively pursued

Exploration of risk assessment without genetic testing

---

Genetic counselors may ask the family to consider how they would feel if the test result is positive, negative, or inconclusive. The process of thinking through the possibilities may help prepare the family for an actual result. Genetic counselors make the family aware of the options to accept, decline, or defer the testing.[1,8,9]

Some genetic tests are marketed to nongenetics clinicians or have recently become available on a direct to consumer basis. Concerns exist about these approaches to testing among those in the medical community because pretest and posttest informed consent and counseling may be absent or limited. Therefore, testing of children in particular is best performed in a medical facility with the participation of a supervising physician, a genetic counselor, and/or other professionals trained in cancer genetics.[9]

## RESULT DISCLOSURE

It is helpful to provide genetic test results in person when possible, given that genetic testing is complex and can have implications for the individual tested as well as family members. This allows for a more detailed discussion of the result and the family's feelings regarding the result. In disclosing a genetic test result, the genetic counselor provides interpretation of the result while at the same time providing support to the family's reaction to the result. A discussion of the accuracy, sensitivity, and specificity of the result is a key element of results disclosure. Parents of children who test positive for a cancer predisposition syndrome should be informed of how the result affects the medical management of their child. Consensus statements and guidelines for some cancer syndromes can be found in the literature and through various cancer organizations such as the American Cancer Society, the National Comprehensive Cancer Network, and the American Gastroenterological Association. If the result causes concern for new clinical features that the patient is not currently experiencing, then referrals to medical professionals should be made as is appropriate.[1,8] In some cases, consensus guidelines are not available, and customized plans may need to be developed. This may involve collaboration between genetics clinicians, oncologists, and other specialists.

Having a positive test result means that a genetic mutation in a gene known to cause a cancer syndrome has been found. Once this occurs, it is important to revisit the pedigree to determine others in the family who may be at risk and encourage the family to inform those relatives. The genetic counselor can assist families in this task by providing letters of explanation or by being available for discussions with those family members. In some cases, if a family is not willing to inform the family members, the genetic counselor must consider his/her duty to warn with input from the ethics committee at the facility. For more information regarding the ethical and legal issues involved in cancer genetic testing, see Chapter 8.

When no disease-causing mutation is identified, the genetic counselor explains the residual risk that remains. Testing for other genetic syndromes may be considered for more information. In some cases, a variant in a cancer predisposition gene is found, but the clinical impact of the genetic variant is not known. This is called a variant of uncertain significance (VUS). Other times, no disease-causing variant is identified in a cancer predisposition gene, but the family and medical history strongly suggest a cancer syndrome. A genetic counselor may make medical management recommendations for a patient or a family based on medical and family history, even in the absence of a positive genetic set result. These are possibilities that should be reviewed in the informed consent process so that families are not surprised when an uninformative negative result or an inconclusive result (VUS) occur.[1,8]

## PSYCHOSOCIAL ASSESSMENT AND SUPPORT

The process of psychosocial assessment and support occurs throughout the genetic counseling and testing process. The first meeting includes a discussion of the reason a family may be interested in genetic testing. The genetic counselor helps normalize a family's feelings of worry, fear, frustration, confusion, anger, etc., as they are common emotions experienced by families with a child with cancer. The process also includes discussion of how a family may feel or cope when a result is available. The whole process of being referred for a cancer genetic test can be stress provoking for families. Anticipating the appointment, reviewing the family and medical history, reviewing risks for cancer in the family, making a decision about testing, waiting for the results of testing, and the responsibility of informing other family members can all be stress-inducing aspects of the process. There are many sources of support available for families. Many cancer support groups exist at local medical centers, and there is a variety of online resources. One online support service is the American Cancer Society, which has a section on children and cancer.[10] Other sources are tumor or syndrome specific. Genetic counselors can help families locate the resources most appropriate for each family. These sources may help a family identify useful versus harmful coping strategies. The genetic counselor may perform a more formal assessment to determine how a person is coping if it seems a person is experiencing more difficulty than is usual. In this case, referral to a mental health specialist may occur.[1,8] See Box 3.2 for an overview of the components of a genetic counseling session.

## REFERRAL INDICATIONS FOR GENETIC COUNSELING

There are several barriers to identifying patients and families who should be referred for genetic counseling when a child has cancer in the family. One very understandable barrier is the focus on the immediate health of the child rather than the family history or even past medical history. Another barrier is that many families have limited knowledge of their family histories. However, the personal and family histories are the keys to appropriate referrals. When there is a family history of

## BOX 3.2
### Elements of Pediatric Cancer Genetic Counseling Session

| | |
|---|---|
| Contracting | Establishment of mutual agenda for appointment between family and genetic counselor |
| Medical history | Medical history intake, tailored to cancer setting |
| Family history | Family history intake, tailored to cancer setting |
| Risk assessment | Determination of whether features present in medical/family history are suggestive of cancer predisposition syndrome |
| Education | Education focused on suspected condition(s) and genetic testing options |
| Genetic testing informed consent | Discussion of benefits, risks, limitations, and possible outcomes of genetic testing |
| Result disclosure | Discussion of genetic test result, including interpretation as well as implications for the patient and his/her relatives |
| Psychosocial assessment and counseling | Assessment of how the family is coping, followed by provision of appropriate support. If more extensive support is needed, mental health referral may be indicated |

several relatives with cancer on one side of the family, the child has had more than one type of cancer, or the child has other clinical features of a syndrome, a referral for genetics evaluation is appropriate. One source of more information about referrals is a practice guideline published by the American College of Medical Genetics with the subtitle "Referral Indications for Cancer Predisposition Assessment."[11] This source is for all cancers, adult and some pediatric cancers, and includes tables where specific types of cancer are listed as well as the other factors to regard when considering a referral. For instance, Box 3.1 of this guideline indicates that any person with a brain tumor or leukemia under age 18 years of age who has café au lait macules, parents who are related to one another, a family history of Lynch syndrome–associated cancer, a second primary tumor, or a sibling with a childhood cancer should be referred. A source more specific to pediatric cancer that includes a detailed table of cancers that can present in childhood as well as possible corresponding syndromes can be found in Knapke et al.[12] For example, this table lists hepatoblastoma and Wilm's tumor as possible associations with Beckwith-Wiedemann syndrome. The table also lists the genes involved, inheritance pattern, other possible clinical features, and recommended cancer monitoring. Anyone with a family history of a known inherited cancer syndrome or mutation in a cancer predisposition gene should be referred for genetic counseling.

The best way to find a genetic counselor is to consult the NSGC (www.NSGC.org), which includes a "Find a Genetic Counselor" feature. The feature allows for a search by location and specialty. Alternatively, a medical geneticist practicing in cancer genetics can be found through the American Society of Medical Genetics (ASMG).[13] The ASMG website includes a "Find Genetic Services" feature. Patients will benefit from the time and attention of these specialized service providers for the treatment and management of cancer.

## REFERENCES

1. Schneider K. *Counseling about Cancer: Strategies for Genetic Counseling.* 3rd ed. New York: Wiley-Blackwell; 2012.
2. *Genetic Counselor's Scope of Practice.* In: *National Society of Genetic Counselor's General NSGC Member Discussion Page;* 2016. Available at: http://www.nsgc.org/.
3. The National Society of Genetic Counselors' Definition Task Force, Resta R, Biesecker BB, et al. A new definition of genetic counseling: National Society of Genetic Counselors' Task Force Report. *J Genet Couns.* 2006;15(2):77–83.
4. Accredited Program. In: *Accreditation Council for Genetic Counseling;* 2017. Available at: http://gceducation.org/Pages/Accredited-Programs.aspx.
5. Professional Status Survey 2016. In: *National Society of Genetic Counselors Website.* Available at: http://www.nsgc.org/page/whoaregeneticcounselors.
6. Robson M, Bradbury A, Arun B, et al. American Society of Clinical Oncology policy statement update: genetic and genomic testing for cancer susceptibility. *J Clin Oncol.* 2006;24(31):5091–5097.
7. Robson M, Storm C, Weitzel J, Wollins D, Offit K. American Society of Clinical Oncology policy statement update: genetic and genomic testing for cancer susceptibility. *J Clin Oncol.* 2015;33(31):3660–3667.
8. Riley B, Culver J, Skrzynia C, et al. Essential elements of genetic cancer risk assessment, counseling, and testing: updated recommendations of the National Society of Genetic Counselors. *J Genet Couns.* 2011;21(2):151–161.
9. Robson M, Storm C, Weitzel J, Wollins D, Offit K. American Society of Clinical Oncology policy statement update: genetic and genomic testing for cancer susceptibility. *J Clin Oncol.* 2010;28(5):893–901.

10. Children and Cancer. In: *American Cancer Society*. Available at: http://www.cancer.org/treatment/childrenandcancer/index.

11. Hampel H, Bennett R, Buchanan A, Pearlman R, Wiesner GA. Practice guideline from the American College of Medical Genetics and Genomics and the National Society of Genetic Counselors: referral indications for cancer predisposition assessment. *Genet Med*. 2015;1:70–87.

12. Knapke S, Zelley K, Nichols K, Kohlmann W, Schiffman J. Identification, management, and evaluation of children with cancer-predisposition syndromes. In: *Am Soc Clin Oncol Educ Book*; 2012:576–584.

13. Find Genetic Services. American College of Medical Genetics Professional Website. Available at: https://www.acmg.net/ACMG/Find_Genetic_Services/ACMG/.

# CHAPTER 4

# Cancer Genetics and Biology

THERESA V. STRONG, PhD

**OVERVIEW**

Cancer development is a multistep process in which cells must acquire certain characteristics to circumvent the inherent controls on abnormal cell proliferation and expansion. This chapter will review factors contributing to the initiation of tumor development, as well as the biologic hallmarks necessary for cancer cells to reach a fully malignant state.

## GENETICS OF TUMOR INITIATION AND PROGRESSION—DEFINING THE GENOMIC LANDSCAPE OF PEDIATRIC TUMORS

Cancer arises from a progressive accumulation of mutations and genomic alterations in normal tissue progenitor and stem cells, resulting in malignant transformation. Both intrinsic and extrinsic factors contribute to the accumulation of mutations and genomic changes. Mutations occur as a natural consequence of repeated cell division—although the DNA is replicated with high fidelity, given the size of the genome and the number of cell divisions necessary for organ development and maintenance, random errors are inevitable. The highly repetitive nature of many sequences in the human genome also contributes to errors. "Slippage" during DNA synthesis may introduce small insertions and deletions, and amplifications, deletions, and translocations can be promoted by short stretches of homology found across the genome. Normal cellular processes contribute to the mutation load as well, because the natural by-products of metabolism, such as reactive oxygen species, can cause DNA damage. Extrinsic factors also play an important role in cancer development and include exposure to radiation, carcinogens, and other environmental factors that increase cancer risk over the lifetime of an individual. Finally, while the majority of cancers, including pediatric cancers, are the result of acquired mutations, pathogenic germline mutations greatly increase cancer risk and are estimated to underlie ~10% of pediatric cases, disproportionately contributing to adrenocortical tumors, osteosarcoma, and acute lymphocytic leukemia.[1,2]

Next-generation sequencing methods have allowed the numerous genetic changes that accompany transformation to be delineated in greater detail. Point mutations, copy number alterations (amplifications and deletions), chromosomal rearrangements, loss or gain of entire chromosomes (aneuploidy), extrachromosomal DNA, and epigenetic changes can all contribute to the altered genetic makeup of cancer cells. Fully defining the molecular landscape of pediatric tumors is important not only for advancing the understanding of cancer development and progression, but also for improving the precision of diagnosis, prognosis, and treatment. The Cancer Genome Atlas (TCGA)[3] is a multiyear collaborative project supported by the National Institutes of Health to understand the genomic changes in more than 30 types of cancer. This project has generated a tremendous amount of data and has revealed characteristic differences in genomic changes across tumor types and subclasses. Although some cancers found in the pediatric population are represented in this effort, most of the cancers selected for TCGA analysis are predominantly found in adult populations. To complement these efforts, a pediatric-specific genome project has been developed: The St. Jude-Washington University Pediatric Cancer Genome Project.[4,5] This effort is not only defining the genomic landscape for common pediatric cancers, such as lymphoblastic leukemias, medulloblastoma, Ewing sarcoma, and neuroblastoma, but also investigating the underlying genetic basis of typically adult tumors, such as melanoma, which sometime occur in children and adolescents. The last 5 years have generated a wealth of knowledge in this regard, providing insight into the origins, progression, and recurrence of both rare and common pediatric cancers.[4–6]

Although a review of the findings to date of the Pediatric Cancer Genome Project is beyond the scope of this chapter, it is apparent that the well-described mechanisms of adult cancer initiation (e.g., point mutations in oncogenes and tumor suppressors, amplifications and deletions, aneuploidy, rearrangements/translocations, and epigenetic changes) are all at play to a greater or lesser degree across the different pediatric cancers. Furthermore, the molecular characteristics and the underlying genomic alterations of pediatric cancers correlate with their cell of origin. Among the changes found at the nucleotide level, point mutations in protooncogenes render normal genes capable of promoting aberrant and continued proliferation, and mutations in known oncogenes such as *NRAS*, *KRAS*, and *BRAF* are among the most frequent changes found in pediatric cancer. Similarly, mutations in tumor suppressor genes, whose normal role is to suppress abnormal cellular growth, also constitute an important molecular alteration, and mutations in *TP53*, the most commonly mutated gene in all cancers, is also the most common mutation found in pediatric cancers. Overall, however, pediatric cancers have lower rates of point mutations at diagnosis compared to adult cancers. Chromosome rearrangements may be particularly relevant for pediatric leukemia, renal cancer, and rhabdomyosarcoma. These rearrangements frequently result in the generation of an oncogenic fusion protein or overexpression of an oncogene, and they may provide rational targets for therapeutic development. Epigenetic changes, including chemical modification of DNA (e.g., methylation and hydroxymethylation) as well as modification of the histone proteins around which DNA is packaged, do not change the actual DNA sequence but do lead to stable changes in gene expression that impact tumor development and progression. Compared with adult tumors, pediatric cancers demonstrate a high mutation frequency in genes that encode epigenetic regulators, and these changes may be particularly important in high-grade glioma, T cell lymphoblastic leukemia, and medulloblastoma.[7]

In the aggregate, studies of the cancer genome and epigenome are providing a clearer picture of the initiating events and genetic drivers of pediatric cancers, as well as defining the changes that allow progressively more aggressive clones to develop and expand. Genome instability is a defining feature of cancer cells, and it generates the intratumoral diversity that can then expedite the development of features necessary for tumor progression. Genomic instability and tumor heterogeneity also complicate the development of effective targeted therapies, as emergence of treatment-resistant subclones poses a challenging problem.[8] Despite these challenges, however, genomics-driven precision medicine has already taken a foothold in the management of pediatric cancers and holds great promise for the future.[9]

## BIOLOGIC HALLMARKS OF CANCER DEVELOPMENT

During progression, cancer cells must acquire certain capabilities to ensure survival and continued expansion. Six key "hallmarks" of cancer development have been described by Hanahan and Weinberg.[10,11] These hallmarks include sustaining proliferative signaling, evading growth suppressors, resisting cell death, enabling replicative immortality, inducing angiogenesis, and activating invasion and metastasis. Each of these traits marks the evolution of cancer through a complex, multistep process. These changes take place in the presence of normal cells, which are recruited and induced to actively support the acquisition of the hallmarks. Progress in understanding the contribution of each of these components can suggest new approaches to cancer prevention and treatment.

### Sustaining Abnormal Proliferation

A fundamental trait of cancer cells is the ability to maintain proliferation. Mutation of normal, growth-promoting protooncogenes represents the most straightforward way to achieve this goal. Mutations in protooncogenes may render the encoded protein permanently activated, capable of ignoring the signals that would normally trigger inactivation. Protooncogenes relevant in pediatric cancers include those that play a role in signal transduction (*NRAS*, *KRAS*, *BRAF*) and transcription (*MYC*, *RUNX1*, *ETV6*), among others.

In addition to activating the oncogenes mentioned above, additional genetic alterations may enhance and sustain abnormal proliferation. For example, the aberrant production and release of growth factors or changes to growth factor receptor pathways to enhance responsiveness or completely deregulate signaling can promote proliferation. These changes may allow proliferation that is independent of the usual growth factor requirements. For example, acquisition of activating mutations and/or amplification and overexpression of growth factor receptor genes (such as those encoding the epidermal growth factor [EGF] receptor and fibroblast growth factor [FGF] receptor) allow the cell to become hyperresponsive to otherwise limited growth factor ligand concentrations or to proliferate in the absence of the ligand entirely. Modification of normal negative feedback loops to render them less effective is another method by which proliferation can be promoted and sustained.

Reprogramming cellular metabolism is another strategy the cancer cells use to sustain proliferation.[12] This adaptation is necessary to allow cancer cells to continue to propagate in a nutrient-poor environment. Tumors markedly increase glucose consumption in comparison to normal, nonproliferating tissue and exhibit enhanced uptake of amino acids. Several major signaling pathways, frequently activated in cancer, contribute to this process. Activating mutations in the phosphoinositide 3-kinase (PI3K)/Akt signaling pathway serve as a master regulator of glucose uptake and glycolysis, while activation of *MYC*, mutation of *RAS* and *SRC* alleles, or deletion of the tumor suppressor RB1 can enhance amino acid uptake. Beyond changes in nutrient acquisition, tumor cells often decouple glycolysis from oxidative phosphorylation, switching largely to a glycolytic pathway for carbon utilization. Although at first pass it may seem counterintuitive that rapidly dividing malignant cells use a less efficient pathway for ATP generation, in fact, the glycolytic intermediates generated by this metabolic shift provide a necessary pool of precursors for the diverse biosynthetic reactions required by proliferating cancer cells.

### Circumventing Growth Suppressors

In addition to acquiring the genetic changes that serve to activate and sustain abnormal proliferation, cancer cells must be able to evade the signals that normally serve to limit excess cell division. Tumor suppressor genes encode proteins that act in a variety of ways to restrict cell growth, allowing progression through the cell cycle only when conditions are favorable. Two major tumor suppressor genes disrupted in a number of tumor types, including pediatric cancers, are the retinoblastoma (*RB1*) and *TP53* (tumor protein p53) genes, encoding the RB and p53 proteins, respectively. *RB1* was the first tumor suppressor gene identified by studying a rare, inherited form of retinoblastoma. Alfred Knudson noted that inheriting one defective copy of *RB1* led to a vastly increased risk of developing retinoblastoma. Despite inheriting the defective allele in all cells, however, only a small number of cells actually initiated tumors. This observation led Knudson to propose that retinoblastoma development required the loss of both copies of *RB1* in a single cell, with the second "hit" coming as a somatic mutation in the normal *RB1* gene. The normal function of the RB1 protein is to integrate cellular signals from internal and external sources and to assess whether to advance the cell

through the cell cycle. The p53 protein has been termed the "guardian of the genome" because it confers stability by sensing cellular stress and DNA damage and halting cell cycle progression until conditions improve. Alternatively, if faced with extensive genomic damage or physiologic stress, p53 normally functions to trigger apoptosis and eliminate the defective cell. Loss or inactivation of p53 represents the most common genetic alteration in cancer and can impact tumor initiation, progression, and metastasis.

In addition to well-characterized tumor suppressors genes, there are several pathways that serve to control proliferation and to maintain tissue homeostasis within confined spaces, and the genes involved in these pathways can serve as noncanonical tumor suppressors. Chief among these are the signals that maintain cells in a quiescent state when they are in contact with other cells, known as contact-mediated growth inhibition. In differentiated tissues, cells interact and communicate with neighboring cells through junctions formed by cell surface adhesion molecules such as E-cadherin, and this network provides a powerful means of controlling growth and maintaining tissue integrity. Cellular polarization is also important for maintaining tissue integrity and attenuating proliferation. These three-dimensional cues can override intrinsic cell proliferation signals and restrict the growth of mutated cells, while loss of the molecules that mediate cell-to-cell contact and polarization allows unfettered expansion of transformed cells and disruption of normal tissue architecture.

### Resisting Cell Death

Apoptosis, or programmed cell death, is a normal developmental process to eliminate damaged or unnecessary cells in a controlled manner. A key part of organ development, tissue homeostasis, and immunity, apoptosis serves to eliminate potentially tumorigenic cells as well. Cells experiencing extensive DNA damage or physiologic stress will trigger the apoptotic process through a p53-dependent process. Alternatively, extracellular signals, such as the Fas ligand, can trigger apoptosis in Fas receptor positive cells. To survive and continue to proliferate, cancer cells use a variety of strategies to resist or evade apoptosis. The apoptotic process consists of a cascade of signaling events that culminates in the activation of the proteolytic caspase enzymes, which advance the controlled demolition of the cell. Dysregulation or disruption of the apoptotic pathway can be achieved through loss of p53, inhibition of proapoptotic signals, or overexpression of antiapoptotic molecules. The *BCL-2* family of regulatory proteins acts at several points along the apoptotic pathway to either promote or inhibit apoptosis, and it is the interaction of BCL-2 proteins with each other and the mitochondria that determines the threshold for induction of apoptosis.[13] Overexpression of prosurvival BCL-2 accelerates tumorigenesis and promotes resistance to therapy, while inhibition or loss of proapoptotic family members also enables tumor progression. Targeting the regulation or function of the BCL-2 proteins has emerged as a strategy to enhance the efficacy of conventional cytotoxic agents.

Autophagy is another normal cellular process designed to recycle cellular organelles and nutrients to sustain cellular metabolism and homeostasis. Cells maintain a low level of autophagy as a means to remove damaged proteins and organelles and efficiently recycle the nutrients. Initially thought to play primarily a tumor suppressor role, the process of autophagy can also be hijacked in cancer cells to promote survival in stressful conditions and facilitate continued aggressive growth where it might not be possible otherwise.[14] Autophagy can promote tumor dormancy and may allow cancer cells to survive during treatment, setting the stage for an eventual recurrence. A better understanding of how autophagy serves both tumor-suppressing and tumor-promoting roles is needed to fully exploit this process to control tumor initiation, progression, and recurrence.

### Enabling Replicative Immortality

To achieve unlimited replication, cancer cells must overcome the normal attrition of telomere length that accompanies division of nonimmortalized cells. Telomeres are composed of a six-base pair nucleotide sequence, tandemly repeated hundreds to thousands of times, which protects the ends of chromosomes. Because of the nature of DNA replication, wherein the DNA polymerase cannot replicate the very end of the chromosomal DNA on the lagging strand, telomeres shorten with every cell division. Shortened telomeres mediate end-to-end fusions between chromosomes, which reduce cell viability, trigger crisis, and induce senescence. The cellular enzyme telomerase uses an RNA template to add on the telomere repeat DNA, lengthening telomeres. Although inactive in most normal differentiated cells, telomerase is reexpressed in the vast majority of tumor cells, where it restores telomere length to the point where senescence and/or apoptosis are averted. Residual end-to-end chromosomal fusions, persisting from a period before telomerase activation, may be carried in neoplastic cells and may evolve into chromosome deletions or amplifications as cancer development progresses.

### Inducing Angiogenesis

The growth of solid tumors, like any tissue mass, requires that cells have adequate access to oxygen and nutrients and that they are able to clear waste and carbon dioxide. For tumors to grow beyond approximately $1-2 \, mm^3$ in size, a blood supply must be developed to support metabolic demands. Angiogenesis, the induction of new, tumor-associated vasculature, is thus critical to tumor development. Tumors must be able to induce an "angiogenic switch" to coax the proliferation of normally quiescent vasculature endothelial cells. Tumor neovasculature development is a complex process that involves a variety of cell types and signaling pathways. Direct effects on vascular endothelial cells or their bone-marrow derived precursors are key to the process, and vascular endothelial growth factor A (VEGF-A) is a critical molecule orchestrating the development of new blood vessels through its actions on these cells. VEGF is upregulated under conditions of hypoxia, inflammation, and oncogenic signaling, which are commonly found in tumors. Additional proangiogenic and antiangiogenic factors secreted by the tumor, as well as cancer-associated fibroblasts (CAFs) and immune cells, include angiopoietins, EGF, transforming growth factors, platelet-derived growth factor, and thrombospondin-1. Under hypoxic conditions, the balance of proangiogenic and antiangiogenic factors switches in favor of angiogenesis, and the signals coordinate to encourage the recruitment, proliferation, and differentiation of endothelial cells into functional vessels. However, vascular development in tumors is far from the precise process in normal development; tumor vasculature is typically disorganized and exhibits poor structural integrity with increased permeability. The density and pattern of neovascularization also shows diversity, with some tumor types characterized by hypovascularization, while others exhibit dense vascularization. The timing of induction of angiogenesis can vary in tumor development, with some early, premalignant lesions already exhibiting robust blood supply. Regardless of the density, integrity, and timing, the new vasculature provides a venue to deliver the necessary oxygen and nutrients to cancer cells and also provides a means for the next step in the clinical progression of tumors—metastasis.

### Activating Invasion and Metastasis

A number of steps are needed for solid tumors to invade and disseminate beyond the primary tumor mass.[15] Cancer cells from solid tumors must be able to survive without cell-to-cell contact, acquire migratory ability, break through the basement membrane, enter the bloodstream, transit through blood and lymphatic vessels, adhere to vessel walls at a distant site, penetrate through the vessel in a process termed "extravasation," and finally, begin to divide and colonize the distant site, establishing a secondary tumor. To successfully perform this series of steps, cancer cells undergo a major shift in gene expression toward a developmental regulatory program, termed "epithelial to mesenchymal transition" (EMT). Activation of an EMT transcriptional program through a set of transcriptional factors, including Snail, Slug, and Twist, results in loss of E-cadherin expression to allow the tumor cell to detach from its neighbors and the surrounding extracellular matrix (ECM). The trascriptional changes also direct changes in morphology to a more spindle-like morphology, and increased motility to facilitate transit. Upregulation of expression of alternative adherens molecules, such as N-cadherin, is consistent with an increased migratory capacity, reminiscent of embryonic development. Additionally, cells undergoing EMT secrete proteases that degrade the basement membrane and allow access to the bloodstream. Once residing at the distant metastatic site, tumor cells may revert back to a less invasive state through the reverse, mesenchymal to epithelial transition. Although the EMT reprogramming is perhaps the most well-described method of achieving metastatic spread, other programs of invasion are apparent in nonepithelial tumor types. For example, gliomas rarely escape the brain but have a highly invasive phenotype, invading normal brain tissue by following vascular and nerve tracks. These cells commandeer chloride and potassium ion channels to drastically alter their cell volume and navigate the narrow spaces of the brain. It is likely that additional, alternative strategies of tumor spreading are routinely used by cancer cells, and a better understanding of all of the possible routes of metastasis will suggest new approaches to intervention.

## THE ROLE OF THE TUMOR MICROENVIRONMENT

As has been noted, tumors are not composed purely of cancerous cells but rather represent a complex tissue that incorporates noncancerous stromal and immune cells, which play important supporting and tumor-promoting roles. The tumor microenvironment (TME) is composed of CAFs, vascular endothelial cells, pericytes, and innate and adaptive immune cells, as well as their associated molecules. The TME can act as a critical regulator of cancer progression and metastasis, and cancer cells actively reprogram their microenvironment to support these processes.[16] Tumors release signals that stimulate normal, resident cells to release growth factors that, in turn, stimulate cancer cell growth, recruit immunosuppressive cells, and promote angiogenesis. CAFs, for example, are an important source of inflammatory cytokines that drive angiogenesis and immune cell recruitment to the tumor. The composition of the ECM also impacts this process by influencing the bioavailability of growth factors. These factors are normally sequestered in pericellular spaces and the ECM, but an array of proteases, sulfatases, and other enzymes can liberate and activate the growth factors, promoting proliferation and invasion. Tumor cells themselves secrete matrix-degrading proteases, but these can also be supplied by stromal cells and infiltrating immune cells such as tumor-associated macrophages (TAMs).

Metabolic changes in the tumor contribute to the perturbations in the microenvironment that encourage tumor growth, promote angiogenesis, and suppress the action of immune cells. Increased extracellular lactate and subsequent acidification of extracellular space attenuates the function of antigen presenting dendritic cells (DCs) and cytotoxic T cells, while polarizing infiltrating macrophages to a tumor-promoting, M2 phenotype. Overexpression of tryptophan-degrading dioxygenases indoleamine2,3-dioxygenase (IDO1 and 2) by cancer cells depletes tryptophan from the microenvironment and promotes apoptosis of effector T cells. Even the way cancer cells die can impact the TME. Cell death by necrosis is common as tumors develop, and it contributes to continued tumor growth by releasing proinflammatory signals into the TME, recruiting the inflammatory cells and setting up an environment that fosters angiogenesis and cancer cell invasion.

A critical and dynamic component of the TME is cells of the immune system. The interaction of cancer cells with the host immune system is a complex, ever-evolving process. Tumors are infiltrated by a broad array of immune cells, including TAMs, monocytes, myeloid-derived suppressor cells, DCs, neutrophils, and lymphocytes such as T-helper (Th) (CD4+) cells, cytotoxic T cells (CD8+), and T regulatory (Treg) cells. Although some of these cells serve to eliminate tumor cells (e.g., DC, Th, CD8+ T cells), overall these cells are protumorigenic and may release inflammatory cytokines (TAMs) or immunosuppressive cytokines (Treg) that impede the induction of effective cytotoxic T cell responses. Infiltrating immune cells (neutrophils, TAMs) also induce inflammation, promote angiogenesis, and support the expansion of stem cell pools. Tumors actively evade immune destruction through a number of strategies, and a "successful" tumor needs to tip the balance of the immune system in favor of a permissive environment. Tumor cells secrete factors that enhance the function of tumor-promoting innate immune cells (e.g., stimulation of macrophages through secretion of colony stimulating factor 1) and suppress the function of antigen presenting cells (DC) and effector T cells (e.g., by secretion of the cytokine IL-10). As cancer cells acquire more mutations and express neoantigens that may be recognized by T cells, a process of "immunoediting" occurs, whereby cells selectively downregulate expression of immunogenic proteins. Tumor cells can also evade destruction by activated T cells by downregulating expression of antigen presenting HLA-1 molecules, effectively "hiding" from these effector cells. Alternatively, or in addition, cancer cells may express inhibitory ligands, such as programmed cell death ligand 1 (PD-L1), which engages T cells through the PD-1 receptor to inhibit T cell proliferation, survival, and effector functions.

As complex as the interactions are, the TME offers new opportunities for therapeutic target development that are being exploited. For example, after years of investigating the fine details of the cancer-immune cells interaction, strategies to modulation of the effector arm of the immune system are showing some encouraging effects and are entering the forefront of cancer therapies.[17] These approaches include treatment with molecules targeting immune checkpoints, which normally restrict effector cell proliferation and function. For example, inhibition of the PD-1/PD-L1 interaction allows propagation of T cell stimulation, resulting in a robust T cell activation and expansion, and more effective tumor cell killing. Additionally, autologous T cells genetically modified to target tumor-associated antigens (chimeric antigen receptor T (CAR-T) cells) have shown impressive results in early stage clinical trials and suggest the potential of immune-based therapies for dramatically impacting patient survival.

## FUTURE DIRECTIONS

As genome sequencing and other "omics" technologies continue to mature and be broadly applied to pediatric cancers, the underlying genetic features and pathway alterations driving pediatric cancer development will be fully appreciated. These insights will continue to refine our understanding of the complex processes that comprise the hallmarks of cancer. Ultimately, the knowledge gained will allow the selection of tailored, targeted treatments based on genomic profile, rather than tissue of origin, toward the goal of treating cancer with reduced toxicity and improved survival and quality of life.

## REFERENCES

1. Parsons DW, Roy A, Yang Y, et al. Diagnostic yield of clinical tumor and germline whole-exome sequencing for children with solid tumors. *JAMA Oncol.* 2016;2:616–624.
2. Zhang J, Walsh MF, Wu G, et al. Germline mutations in predisposition genes in pediatric cancer. *N Engl J Med.* 2015;373:2336–2346.
3. The Cancer Genome Atlas. https://cancergenome.nih.gov.
4. Downing JR, Wilson RK, Zhang J, et al. The Pediatric Cancer Genome Project. *Nat Genet.* 2012;44:619–622.
5. The Pediatric Cancer Genome Project. https://www.stjude.org/research/pediatric-cancer-genome-project.html.
6. Childhood Cancer Genomics (PDQ®) Health Professional Version PDQ Pediatric Treatment Editorial Board. https://www.ncbi.nlm.nih.gov/books/NBK374260/.
7. Huether R, Dong L, Chen X, et al. The landscape of somatic mutations in epigenetic regulators across 1,000 paediatric cancer genomes. *Nat Commun.* 2014;5:3630.
8. Morrissy AS, Garzia L, Shih DJ, et al. Divergent clonal selection dominates medulloblastoma at recurrence. *Nature.* 2016;529:351–357.
9. Mody RJ, Presner JR, Evertt J, et al. Precision medicine in pediatric oncology: lessons learned and next steps. *Pediatr Blood Cancer.* 2017;64:e26288.
10. Hanahan D, Weinberg RA. The hallmarks of cancer. *Cell.* 2000;100:57–70.
11. Hanahan D, Weinberg RA. Hallmarks of cancer: the next generation. *Cell.* 2011;144:646–674.
12. Pavlova NN, Thompson CB. The emerging hallmarks of cancer metabolism. *Cell Metab.* 2016;23:27–47.
13. Czabotar PE, Lessene G, Strasser A, Adams JM. Control of apoptosis by the BCL-2 protein family: implications for physiology and therapy. *Nat Rev Mol Cell Biol.* 2014;15:49–63.
14. White E. The role of autophagy in cancer. *J Clin Invest.* 2015;125:42–46.
15. Talmadge JE, Fidler IJ. AACR centennial series: the biology of cancer metastasis: historical perspective. *Cancer Res.* 2010;70:5649–5669.
16. Hanahan D, Coussens LM. Accessories to the crime: functions of cells recruited to the tumor microenvironment. *Cancer Cell.* 2012;21:309–322.
17. Whiteside TL, Demaria S, Rodriguez-Ruiz ME, et al. Emerging opportunities and challenges in cancer immunotherapy. *Clin Cancer Res.* 2016;22:1845–1855.

# CHAPTER 5

# Genetic Testing Techniques

ALICIA GOMES, MS • BRUCE KORF, MD, PHD

## INTRODUCTION

Genetic testing consists of the analysis of DNA (deoxyribonucleic acid), or in some cases RNA (ribonucleic acid) transcribed from DNA, for variations that are associated with disease or risk of disease. DNA is the molecule responsible for transmission of genetic information in the cell. It consists of a double helix comprised of a sugar-phosphate chain, with the two strands bridged by hydrogen bonding between the four nucleoside bases—adenine (A), guanine (G), cytosine (C), and thymine (T). Base pairing is specific: A always binds with T on the opposite strand, and C binds with G. The order of bases determines the coding sequence, which is copied into a complementary RNA molecule (consisting of a single-stranded ribose-phosphate chain with the same four bases, except that uracil [U] substitutes for thymine). This messenger RNA is then exported to the cytoplasm, where RNA associates with ribosomes to direct the synthesis of proteins, with triplets of bases encoding specific amino acids. The genetic information, consisting of 3.15 billion base pairs of DNA in each haploid genome, is tightly compacted into the cell nucleus and divided into 23 chromosomes, including 22 nonsex chromosomes (autosomes), and the X and Y sex chromosomes (Fig. 5.1).

The essence of genetics, and the basis for genetic testing, is genetic variation. This can occur at multiple levels, from abnormalities at the level of the entire chromosome down to changes at the single nucleotide level. In this chapter we will consider the various methods available for detection of this genetic variation, along with pitfalls in interpretation of the results of genetic tests.

## SOMATIC VERSUS GERMLINE GENETIC VARIATION

Every individual begins with a single pluripotent zygote that replicates into over 37 trillion differentiated cells. If a genetic variant is present in the zygote, it will be replicated in every cell, including future germ cells. This is classified as a **germline variant**. Germline variants can be without phenotypic effect or can result in phenotypes that may include specific genetic syndromes and disorders. Germline variants are associated with a risk of transmission to future offspring and can be transmitted in either a recessive or a dominant pattern. Germline variants can be identified in any tissue specimen, as the variant is represented in all cells in the body. Peripheral blood is commonly used for germline genetic testing, as it is readily accessible for collection and provides an ample source of genetic material within white blood cells.

Genetic variants may also be acquired by a new mutation in somatic cells. Such postzygotic mutations result in the phenomenon of **mosaicism**. The phenotypic effects of a mosaic variant depend on the developmental stage at which the mutation occurred, the gene involved, and the cell lines affected. Mosaicism can result in a fully expressed phenotype, a mildly expressed phenotype if only a small proportion of cells are involved, or a phenotype confined to a single region of the body. In some cases, a mutation occurs during germ cell development, resulting in **germline mosaicism**; in such cases, there is no phenotype, but genetic transmission to multiple offspring may occur (Fig. 5.2).

Throughout life, additional mutations can be acquired somatically, either spontaneously or because of exposure to mutagenic agents, such as chemicals or radiation. This may have no phenotypic effect, but in some cases mutation of a tumor suppressor gene or oncogene can result in malignancy.

## CYTOGENETIC VERSUS MOLECULAR GENETIC TESTING

Chromosomes were discovered in the 1840s in plant cells by Karl Wilhelm von Nageli. The identification of mitosis in animal cells by Walther Flemming in the 1880s paved the way to recognition of the chromosome as a unit of inheritance in the cell. Routine human cytogenetic analysis was developed in the mid-1950s when it was discovered that hypotonic treatment could be used to swell cultured cells, spreading chromosomes at metaphase, the time of greatest condensation, to permit analysis. Subsequent advances included the use of phytohemagglutinin

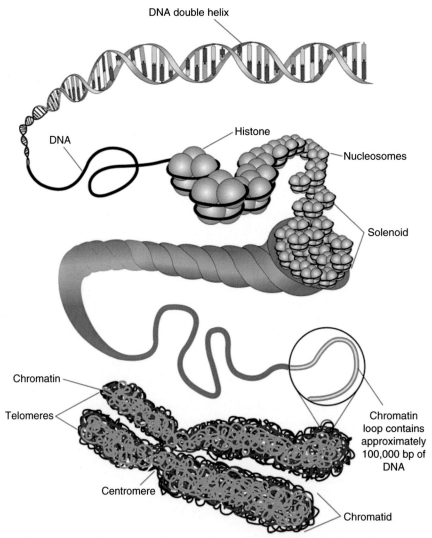

FIG. 5.1 DNA organized within a chromosome. (Courtesy of Jorde LB et al. 2009 Medical Genetics, 4th edn. Elsevier, Edinburgh.)

to stimulate T cell proliferation in peripheral blood cultures and development of staining techniques to elicit characteristic banding patterns that enable precise identification of each chromosome and detection of subtle structural variants. Beginning in the 1980s, fluorescence in situ hybridization (FISH) was developed, enabling detection of specific labeled segments of DNA hybridized to their homologous sequences and consequent detection of deletions or duplications (**copy number variants**). Molecular cytogenetic technologies were further developed in the 2000s with the advent of cytogenomic microarrays, based on hybridization of DNA in a test sample against an array of oligonucleotides on a "chip,"

permitting high-resolution detection of copy number variants down to a few thousand base pairs.

In contrast with these high-level analyses of structural variants or copy number changes, molecular analyses began to be developed to detect variants down to the level of a single nucleotide. Detection of variants at the DNA level has also undergone evolution, including the development of sequencing technologies applicable to specific genes (e.g., Sanger sequencing) and now toward sequencing of the entire genome using massively parallel ("next-generation") technologies. The scale of detection for molecular analysis ranges from the single nucleotide level to an entire gene or group of

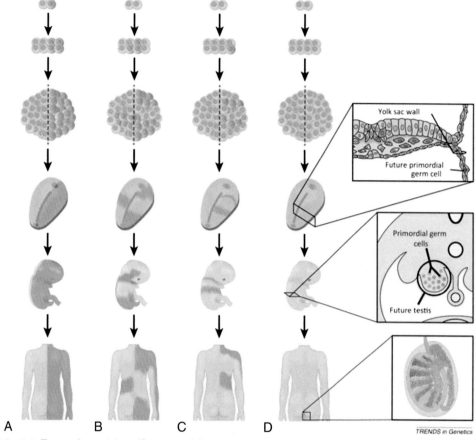

FIG. 5.2 Types of mosaicism. (Courtesy of Campbell I, Shaw C, Stankiewicz P, et al. Somatic mosaicism: implications for disease and transmission genetics. *Trends Genet.* July 2015;31(7):382–392.) Examples A-C describe possible phenotypic severity outcomes based on the timing of the mutation during embryogenesis. Example D describes the unique phenomenon of germline mosaicism when a mutation is isolated to a percentage of the primordial germ cells.

genes, forming now a continuum between cytogenetic/cytogenomic to molecular analysis.

## CLASSIFICATION OF GENETIC VARIATION
Genetic variation can extend from the level of the single nucleotide up to the entire chromosome. Table 5.1 provides a classification of the different types of genetic variants.

## CYTOGENETIC ANALYSIS
### Karyotype
#### Methodology
Karyotyping involves analysis of the entire chromosome complement through the microscope. Dividing cells are harvested during metaphase, the time of greatest chromosome condensation, by disruption of the spindle using drugs such as colchicine. Chromosomes are visualized by staining, including the use of special stains to elicit banding patterns (Table 5.2). In general GC-rich regions tend to be gene rich and stain darkly with G-banding, bright with R-banding, and dark with Q-banding[1] (Fig. 5.3).

Karyotyping is able to detect polyploidy, aneuploidy, translocations, inversions, rings, and copy number changes in the size range of 4–6 Mb; smaller copy number changes require the use of molecular cytogenetic techniques.[1]

#### *Types of variants detected*
- Polyploidy
- Monosomies/trisomies
- Inversions
- Translocations
- Large microdeletions/duplications

**TABLE 5.1**
**Classification of Genetic Variants**

| Variant Type | Definition | Example |
|---|---|---|
| **CHROMOSOME LEVEL** | | |
| Polyploidy | An entire extra set of chromosomes | Triploidy, having three haploid chromosome sets |
| Aneuploidy (monosomy/trisomy) | An entire missing (monosomy) or extra chromosome (trisomy) | Trisomy 21, Turner syndrome |
| Translocation | An exchange of genetic material between two chromosomes. This can be balanced (no missing material) or unbalanced (partial deletions or duplications) | Burkitt's lymphoma due to a translocation of chromosomes 8 and 14: t(8;14)(q24;q32) |
| Inversion | A segment within a chromosome that has been reversed. It may include (pericentric) or not include (paracentric) the centromere | Inversion within chromosome 16 seen in an aggressive subtype of pediatric acute megakaryoblastic leukemia: inv(16)(p13.3q24.3) |
| Copy number variant | Deletion or duplication of DNA segments | 21q11.2 microdeletion associated with DiGeorge syndrome; deletion of multiple exons in dystrophin gene resulting in Duchenne muscular dystrophy |
| **NUCLEOTIDE LEVEL** | | |
| Deletion/duplication | Any combination of loss or gain of one or several nucleotides; a deletion or duplication that is not an integral multiple of three bases results in a frameshift | One base deletion resulting in frameshift |
| Nonsense | A base substitution that creates a new stop signal | C to T change in arginine codon, resulting in stop |
| Missense | A base substitution that alters the amino acid encoded at a specific codon | Sickle cell variant in β-globin |
| Silent | A base substitution that does not alter the amino acid at a codon | A single nucleotide polymorphism common in the general population |
| Splicing variant | A base substitution in an exon or intron that alters RNA splicing | Splice donor variant that results in exon skipping |

**TABLE 5.2**
**Banding Techniques and Stains**

| Banding Technique | Stain | Clinical Application |
|---|---|---|
| G (Giemsa)-banding | Giemsa | Most commonly used for karyotyping. Used as the reference for banding points. Gene-rich regions stain darkly |
| R (reverse)-banding | Acridine orange | Gene-rich bands fluoresce brightly |
| C (centromere)-banding | Giemsa stain with alkali, acid, salt, or heat treatment | Identifies heterochromatin associated with each centromere |
| Q (quinacrine)-banding | Quinacrine | AT-rich regions fluoresce brightly |

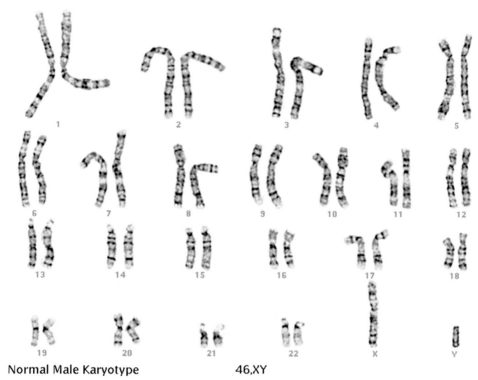

Normal Male Karyotype                     46,XY

FIG. 5.3 Normal male karyotype. (Courtesy of Dr. Fady Mikhail, MD, PhD, FACMG. University of Alabama at Birmingham Cytogenetics Laboratory.)

## Benefits

Within the germline, there are syndromes caused by large structural rearrangements that are known to have an increased predisposition to tumors. Individuals with Down syndrome, associated with trisomy 21, have a 10- to 20-fold risk for acute lymphocytic leukemia, acute myelocytic leukemia, and acute megakaryocytic leukemia.[2] Individuals with Klinefelter syndrome, a condition in males caused by having an extra copy of the X chromosome (XXY sex chromosomes), are at an increased risk for breast cancer, extragonadal germ cell tumors, non-Hodgkin lymphoma, and lung cancer.[3] Individuals with Turner syndrome, caused by having a single copy of the X chromosome in females, have an increased risk for Wilms' tumor, leukemia, gonadal tumors, neurogenic tumors, and uterine tumors in those taking unopposed estrogen.[4]

Karyotypes can be used in somatic cells for treatment and prognosis. Many tumors and cancers acquire chromosomal changes as they progress. A karyotype can be performed on dividing cancer cells to help in classification, as certain chromosomal changes are characteristic of specific cancers.

## Limitations

Chromosome analysis will not identify all genetic anomalies. When a deletion or duplication is smaller than 4–6 Mb in size, the variant may be missed by karyotypic analysis. In addition, chromosomal analysis can be challenging in cancer cells, where morphologic preservation may be less than in somatic cells. Accuracy of chromosomal analysis is also heavily dependent on the skill of the technologist. Lastly, mosaicism may be an important factor, as low level mosaicism may be missed. The number of cells routinely analyzed is dependent on the tissue type, whether the specimen has been cultured, and the purpose of the analysis.

### Fluorescence In Situ Hybridization
### Methodology

Fluorescence In Situ Hybridization (FISH) analysis is performed by denaturing the double-stranded DNA in the fixed chromosomes on a microscope slide. Once denatured, two fluorescently labeled DNA probes are used in combination to analyze each location in question. The first probe serves as a control and hybridizes with DNA on the target chromosome but outside of

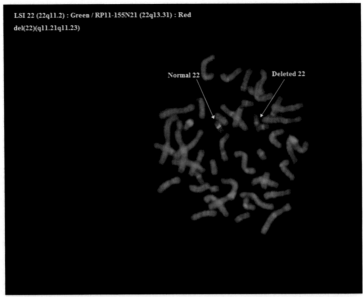

FIG. 5.4 Fluorescence in situ hybridization (FISH) probe notating a deletion on the long arm of chromosome 22. (Courtesy of Dr. Fady Mikhail, MD, PhD, FACMG. University of Alabama at Birmingham Cytogenetics Laboratory.)

the targeted region. The second probe hybridizes to a target location on the individual's DNA sequence. When the sequence is present, the probe will hybridize and fluoresce with a different color than the control probe.

When a deletion is present, the second probe will not hybridize and no fluorescence will be seen. A duplication will result in two fluorescent spots with the test probe (Fig. 5.4).

### Types of variants detected
- Monosomy/trisomy
- Balanced/unbalanced translocations
- Microdeletions/duplications

### Benefits
FISH analysis can be helpful in germline analysis of large deletions and duplications. This testing process has a quick turnaround of typically 2–3 business days. This enables an immediate clinical confirmation in time-sensitive medical situations. FISH is also used in diagnosis and follow-up of cancer. FISH probes have been designed for most common deletions, duplications, and translocations that have been identified in many cancer types where the mutation in question will provide insights into how well the tumor or cancer in question will respond to a certain therapeutic agent. Some laboratories offer probe panels that include several FISH probes for the most common

regions analyzed and offer a simultaneous analysis of the genetic material. FISH analysis can also be very helpful in the identification of mosaicism, as several cells can be analyzed simultaneously in one analysis.

### Limitations
FISH analysis requires an adequately sized tissue sample for analysis. It is also necessary to predetermine the target for analysis; if there is a copy number change outside the target region, it will not be detected.

### Microarray
### Methodology
DNA microarrays can be used to analyze the expression or copy number of multiple genes throughout multiple regions of the genome simultaneously. The following are a list of types of DNA microarrays available and their applications[5]; however, we will only focus on two approaches in this chapter (Table 5.3).

The two most frequently utilized DNA microarray technologies for genotyping are the comparative genomic hybridization (CGH) microarray and the single nucleotide polymorphism (SNP) array. The CGH microarray uses a small plate of glass (chip), typically less than an inch in size. The chip contains a grid consisting of thousands of probes to specific segments within the human genome. The test sample DNA is digested to create fragments and a fluorescent dye is added to the specimen.

---

**TABLE 5.3**
**Microarrays and Applications**

| Microarray Name | Application |
|---|---|
| Gene expression profiling | Observes expression levels of thousands of genes simultaneously. Useful when analyzing the treatment and advancement of diseases and choice of therapeutics |
| Comparative genome hybridization (CGH) | Compares the genetic content of two similar specimens; used to identify copy number changes in a test sample as compared with a reference sample |
| Single nucleotide polymorphism (SNP) | Measures hybridization with oligonucleotide probes that recognize SNPs across the genome; useful in detecting copy number changes or loss of heterozygosity |
| Exon junction array | Uses fewer probes per gene to assess the expression of alternative splicing of a gene in a sample |
| Fusion gene | Detects fusion transcripts resulting from translocations commonly found in cancer specimens for treatment and prognosis |
| Multistranded DNA | Used in the detection of novel drugs that may inhibit the expression of particular genes |
| Bacterial artificial chromosomes (BAC) | Oligonucleotide probes consisting of BACs used to target specific regions of the genome for copy number analysis |

---

The sample is combined with a reference DNA sample that has been digested into fragments and labeled with a different fluorescent tag. The combined specimen is separated into single-stranded DNA and washed over the chip of probes so that the specimens can compete with one another to hybridize with the available DNA probes. The results are analyzed by determining the ratio of test DNA to reference DNA at each available probe based on the visible fluorescence.

SNP microarray technology also takes place on a small plate of glass (chip). The chip contains tens of thousands of regions on which unique DNA probes sit to target specific areas of the genome. Each probe contains a small sequence (~25 base pairs) that surrounds an established SNP within the genome. A probe is created to represent each genotype. For example, if there is a SNP that causes the C allele to be replaced by a T:

…..ATGCTGT<u>C</u>TGTTAC……
…..ATGCTGT<u>T</u>TGTTAC……

A probe will be located on the chip with the complementing G allele to hybridize to individuals with the C allele in their DNA sequence, and a separate probe will be located on the chip with the complementing A allele to hybridize to individuals with the T allele in their sequence.

To perform the analysis, DNA is extracted from an individual. The DNA for each locus is denatured, amplified, and digested. Biotin is also added to enable the individual's DNA sample to adhere to a fluorescent marker later in the process. The individual's DNA is washed over the probe-laden chip for >12 h to provide ample opportunity for hybridization between the test

DNA and the probes. The chip is then rinsed to remove the excess DNA that did not hybridize with the regions captured by the probes. A second wash with a fluorescent marker is then added to adhere to the individual DNA that has hybridized to the probes. Any excess stain that does not bind to a DNA sample is removed. A laser then scans the reaction to measure the amount of fluorescence that is created at each SNP region. As a probe is available for each possible genotype for each SNP location, individuals who are heterozygous or homozygous for a specific location can be identified. Further analysis for copy number variation is performed by normalizing the fluorescence produced by the individual's sample to a reference sample. Copy number loss or gain, uniparental disomy, and large regions of homozygosity can be visualized using this technology (Fig. 5.5).

*Types of variants detected*
- Monosomy/trisomy
- Unbalanced translocations
- Microdeletions/duplications
- Large deletions/duplications

*Benefits*
Many genetic testing laboratories use a microarray technology to identify copy number changes for the genes analyzed in their panels. This can be very helpful for patients presenting with a phenotype that overlaps with several possible genetic etiologies. An array allows for the simultaneous analysis of multiple genes for identification of copy number variants.

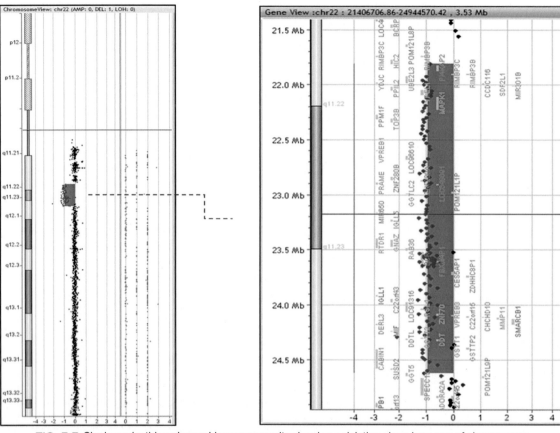

FIG. 5.5 Single nucleotide polymorphism array results showing a deletion along long arm of chromosome 22. TypeIII distal 22q11.2 microdeletion (~2.8 Mb in size) that spans the *SMARCB1* gene (MIM: 611867). (Courtesy of Dr. Fady Mikhail, MD, PhD, FACMG. University of Alabama at Birmingham Cytogenetics Laboratory.)

Microarray-based platforms are highly sensitive in detecting copy number variations ranging from a single exon to aneuploidy/polyploidy. This can be very helpful in classifying a tumor and in guiding treatment and prognosis.

### Limitations

Microarray technology can be expensive when compared with other technologic approaches that could be used to identify similar alterations. Microarray technology is also limited in the mutational spectrum that can be identified. While SNP arrays can be used to identify various forms of copy number change, it is unable to identify copy number variants smaller than ~80kb. Balanced translocations are also not identified, which is a limitation in cancer diagnosis. Mosaicism detection is also a limitation of microarrays because a mutation present in fewer than 20%–30% of the cells may be missed by this approach.[6] This can be important when dealing with a starting material containing a mixed etiology or if an individual only harbors a mutation in a small percentage of their cell lines.

## Multiplex Ligation-Dependent Probe Amplification

### Methodology

Multiplex Ligation-dependent Probe Amplification (MLPA) is a polymerase chain reaction (PCR)-based technique that analyzes several loci simultaneously for small copy number changes, usually involving one or several exons. MLPA begins with a denaturation of double-stranded DNA into single strands and hybridization to MLPA probes located at distinct intervals throughout the exons of the gene in question. Each probe consists of two separate oligonucleotides (one at the 5′ and one at the 3′ end) of the interval to be tested. A ligation reaction follows when the adjacent probes are able to hybridize with their target sequences. In addition to the gene-specific oligonucleotides, each probe also includes a universal primer sequence that enables a simultaneous PCR reaction to take place. All of the ligated probes in the assay amplify the ligated probes and then each PCR product is separated using capillary electrophoresis. The products are then analyzed by measuring the fluorescence produced by the amount of PCR product that is made after the amplification compared with control peaks that assess the quality of the amplification step and standardizes the amount of DNA present at each locus (Fig. 5.6).

### Types of variants detected
- Single/multiexon deletions
- Single/multiexon duplications

### Benefits
MLPA is analyzed and interpreted by the presence of PCR product measured in the patient sample in comparison with control peaks. MLPA analysis can detect homozygous or hemizygous deletions and duplications. The probes used for MLPA analysis can detect copy number changes involving as few as 60 nucleotides, enabling identification of single exon deletions. MLPA technology is useful in cancer genetics for both somatic and germline testing. Many germline tumor and cancer predisposition syndromes present with a spectrum of mutations, including copy number variants. It is important to review the mutational spectrum known for each condition in consideration and compare this with the testing options available for each laboratory's testing strategy.

### Limitations
MLPA is only capable of identifying copy number variations. Furthermore, identifying a deletion or duplication will not define the exact break points of the mutation; MLPA can only certify that a deletion or duplication is present. If a variant has break points that extend past the last probe deleted in an assay but end before the next probe analyzed, it cannot be concluded where the deletion starts/stops within this region. MLPA is also gene/region-specific. For example, if an MLPA analysis concludes that there is a duplication of all the probes in the assay, it cannot be determined if the duplication is really due to a chromosomal anomaly or a duplication involving multiple genes. Additional technology must be used

to define these details. Lastly, MLPA has limited ability to identify a mosaic deletion/duplication if the variant is present in fewer than 30% of the cells analyzed.[7]

### Sanger Sequencing
#### Methodology
Sanger sequencing is a targeted sequencing technique that uses oligonucleotide primers to seek out specific DNA regions. Sanger sequencing begins with denaturation of the double-stranded DNA. The single-stranded DNA is then annealed to oligonucleotide primers and elongated using a mixture of deoxynucleotide triphosphates (dNTPs), which provide the needed arginine (A), cytosine (C), tyrosine (T), and guanine (G) nucleotides to build the new double-stranded structure. In addition, a small quantity of chain-terminating dideoxynucleotide triphosphates (ddNTPs) for each nucleotide is included. The sequence will continue to extend with dNTPs until a ddNTP attaches. As the dNTPs and ddNTPs have an equal chance of attaching to the sequence, each sequence will terminate at varying lengths.

Each ddNTP (ddATP, ddGTP, ddCTP, ddTTP) also includes a fluorescent marker. When a ddNTP is attached to the elongating sequence, the base will fluoresce based on the associated nucleotide. By convention, A is indicated by green fluorescence, T by red, G by black, and C by blue. A laser within the automated machine used to read the sequence detects a fluorescent intensity that is translated into a "peak." When a heterozygous variant occurs within a sequence, loci will be captured by two fluorescent dyes of equal intensity. When a homozygous variant is present, the expected fluorescent color is replaced completely by the new base pair's color (Fig. 5.7).

### Types of variants detected
- Silent
- Missense
- Nonsense
- Truncating
- Deletion
- Insertion
- Splicing

### Benefits
Sanger sequencing is a robust testing strategy able to determine whether a point mutation or small deletion/duplication is present. It has been widely used for several decades in many settings, including defining the mutational spectrum of a tumor as well as identifying a constitutional variant in diagnostic testing. Primers can be created to cover several regions (amplicons) to cover any size region of interest.

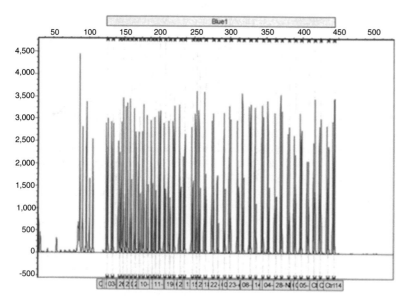

| | Probe Name | Bin Size | Height Ratio |
|---|---|---|---|
| 1 | 01-TBX1 | 177.7 | 1.219 |
| 2 | 02-TBX1 | 253.0 | 1.162 |
| 3 | 03-DGCR8 | 148.6 | 1.184 |
| 4 | 04-SNAP29 | 371.8 | 0.896 |
| 5 | 05-LZTR1 | 417.7 | 1.395 |
| 6 | 06-PPIL2 | 408.6 | 1.000 |
| 7 | 07-GNAZ | 143.7 | 0.895 |
| 8 | 08-exon1 | 336.3 | 0.341 |
| 9 | 09-exon1 | 311.7 | 0.500 |
| 10 | 10-exon2b | 195.3 | 0.459 |
| 11 | 11-exon2b | 215.1 | 0.419 |
| 12 | 12-exon3 | 160.4 | 0.474 |
| 13 | 13-exon3 | 257.9 | 0.454 |
| 14 | 14-exon4 | 354.2 | 0.428 |
| 15 | 15-exon4 | 265.9 | 0.490 |
| 16 | 16-exon5 | 190.6 | 0.521 |
| 17 | 17-exon5 | 208.7 | 0.496 |
| 18 | 18-exon6 | 283.8 | 0.390 |
| 19 | 19-exon6 | 230.3 | 0.445 |
| 20 | 20-exon7 | 363.9 | 0.406 |
| 21 | 21-exon7 | 184.4 | 0.497 |
| 22 | 22-exon8 | 293.0 | 0.460 |
| 23 | 23-exon8 | 318.6 | 0.472 |
| 24 | 24-exon9 | 172.6 | 0.491 |
| 25 | 25-exon9 | 247.7 | 0.574 |
| 26 | 26-SNRPD3 | 166.2 | 0.838 |
| 27 | 27-SEZ6L | 276.6 | 1.056 |
| 28 | 28-NIPSNAP1 | 390.4 | 0.835 |
| 29 | Ctrl01 | 126.6 | 1.032 |
| 30 | Ctrl02 | 134.1 | 0.984 |
| 31 | Ctrl03 | 154.5 | 1.021 |
| 32 | Ctrl04 | 201.3 | 1.005 |
| 33 | Ctrl05 | 221.4 | 1.120 |
| 34 | Ctrl06 | 236.2 | 1.233 |
| 35 | Ctrl07 | 300.6 | 0.908 |
| 36 | Ctrl08 | 328.4 | 1.010 |
| 37 | Ctrl09 | 346.2 | 0.923 |
| 38 | Ctrl10 | 381.9 | 1.058 |
| 39 | Ctrl11 | 399.0 | 0.878 |
| 40 | Ctrl12 | 425.9 | 1.061 |
| 41 | Ctrl13 | 436.2 | 0.839 |
| 42 | Ctrl14 | 444.6 | 1.177 |

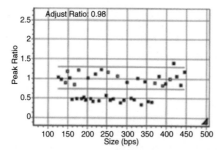

**FIG. 5.6** Graphic representation of a Multiplex Ligation-dependent Probe Amplification (MLPA) analysis showing a multi exon deletion. (Courtesy of Dr. Ludwine Messiaen, PhD, FACMG. University of Alabama at Birmingham Molecular Genomics Laboratory.)

### Limitations

Although one could use individual Sanger sequencing reactions to cover any desired region, this testing approach can be costly when compared with other multiplex testing systems. Therefore, most currently available Sanger sequencing tests are gene-specific or analyze a small subset of genes. Sanger sequencing is able to identify mosaic mutations including as low as 20% of the cells, but Sanger sequencing is not precisely quantifiable. For example, one cannot conclude if a mutation is present in 25% versus 40% of cells based on peak sizes; additional testing strategies must be used for quantification.

### Next-Generation Sequencing
#### Methodology

"Next-generation" sequencing (NGS) is a high-throughput technology that enables simultaneous sequencing of multiple DNA segments in a sample. This analysis is accomplished by parallel sequencing of small fragments

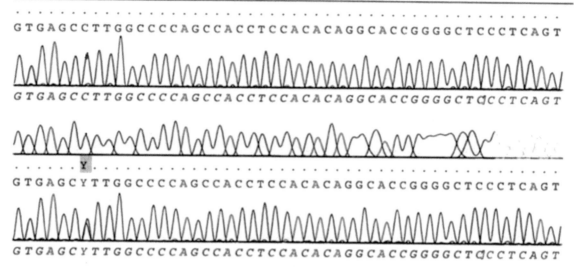

FIG. 5.7 Electropherogram from Sanger sequencing of a nucleotide change from C to T (mutation noted with a Y) compared to sequencing of normal contral samples. This mutation is a heterozygous mutation as both alleles harbor a different nucleotide. (Courtesy of Dr. Ludwine Messiaen, PhD, FACMG. University of Alabama at Birmingham Molecular Genomics Laboratory.)

and aligning these to a reference sequence. Different platforms use different sequencing approaches, with current major platforms summarized in Table 5.4. NGS can be used to sequence the entire complement of DNA in a sample (whole genome sequencing—WGS) or specific segments can be isolated for sequencing. These can include all of the exons (whole exome sequencing—WES), or specific regions of interest, creating "panels" of genes to be sequenced.[8]

### Types of variants detected
- Silent
- Missense
- Nonsense
- Truncating
- Deletion
- Insertion
- Splicing

### Single gene versus panel versus whole exome/genome testing

One major benefit of NGS is the ability to test tens to hundreds to thousands of genes simultaneously. This is especially helpful in testing individuals who present with an ambiguous clinical presentation in which multiple genes could be the underlying cause. Panel-based testing eliminates the time and financial strain required to sequence several individual genes until the

right gene is identified. Panel-based testing is also especially helpful when any of several genes may be known to cause a specific disorder.

NGS testing strategies also produce multiple, individually produced readings of the target area compared with Sanger sequencing, which only provides one aggregated read. This is most beneficial when evaluating for mosaicism. NGS testing becomes a quantitative approach of determining mosaicism by calculating the percentage of individual reads produced with the mutation versus those without the mutation (Fig. 5.8).

NGS can also expand beyond panel testing options, into whole exome or genome sequencing. Whole exome/genome sequencing can be useful when it is suspected that the genetic cause for an individual clinical presentation is not well established and likely unavailable in an individual gene or panel option. Whole exome/genome sequencing can also become helpful when someone has exhausted the panel-based options currently available for a condition and no mutation has been found. Lastly, when an individual presents with a phenotype that overlaps with multiple conditions, a whole exome/genome testing approach can be helpful in examining several genes simultaneously. The choice of whole genome versus exome sequencing depends in part on costs (WGS is significantly more expensive than WES currently) and degree of coverage required. WGS offers the possibility

**TABLE 5.4**
Sequencing: Platform, Target Amplification, Sequencing Platform, and Sequencing Chemistry

| Platform | Target Amplification Technique | Sequencing Platform | Sequencing Chemistry |
|---|---|---|---|
| 454/Roche | On-bead emulsion PCR | Beads are placed in individual wells for sequencing | Uses pyrosequencing by detecting pyrophosphate as it is released when each base pair is added |
| Illumina (MiSeq/HiSeq/NextSeq) | Array-based "Bridge-PCR" | Each targeted DNA region is sequenced within a cluster randomly placed on the surface of a chip | The fluorescence of each base pair is captured as it is added to each amplicon |
| SOLiD | On-bead emulsion PCR | Beads are randomly located on the surface of a chip and each small oligonucleotide is labeled and sequenced in this location | The fluorescence of each base pair is captured as is it added to each amplicon |
| Ion Torrent | On-bead emulsion PCR | Beads are placed in individual wells for isolated sequencing | Detects proton release as each base pair is added |

*PCR*, polymerase chain reaction.

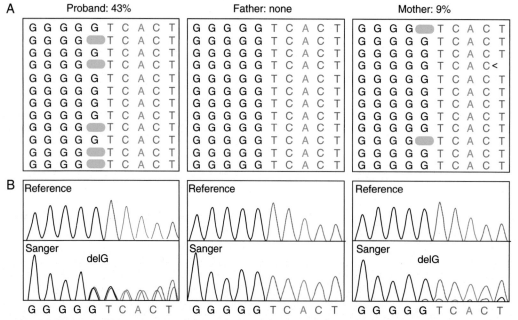

FIG. 5.8 Mosaic JAG1 mutation in maternal blood. **(A)** Next-generation sequencing detects a heterozygous JAG1:c.1499delG (p.G500Vfs*64) mutation in the proband; 9% of mutation load is detected in the mother, and the father is negative for this mutation. **(B)** Sanger sequencing results for this mutation. (Courtesy of Qin L, Wang J, Tian X, Yu H, et al. Detection and quantification of mosaic mutations in disease genes by next-generation sequencing. *J Mol Diagn.* May 2016;18(3):446–453. http://dx.doi.org/10.1016/j.jmoldx.2016.01.002. Epub 2016 Mar 2.)

| TABLE 5.5 Guide to Testing Approaches | | |
|---|---|---|
| **Single Gene (Sanger)** | **Panel Testing (NGS)** | **Whole Exome/Genome (NGS)** |
| An individual has hallmark features that are indicative to one specific condition, which has a single gene associated with the phenotype; specific cancer-related variant is suspected | An individual has some features of a condition in which there are multiple genes that can be associated with the condition or conditions with overlapping presentations; multiple specific genes are tested that can be associated with a particular cancer | An individual presents with clinical features that can overlap several conditions and no specific gene or condition can be pinpointed as a starting point; the entire complement of genetic variants in a tumor needs to be identified |

of detection of pathogenic variants outside the coding region of genes, although validating these as pathogenic can be challenging. Also, the bioinformatic analysis of the very large number of variants found by WGS can be more time-consuming and expensive.

Given the complexities and the unique approaches needed based on each individual's presenting circumstance, it can be difficult to determine what is the best place to start when deciding on a testing approach. Table 5.5 provides a guide that can be considered.

### Limitations

NGS is limited by the analysis and bioinformatics pipeline used to analyze the data. Most NGS testing strategies are limited in their ability to detect copy number variations; however, the size and limits are specific to the bioinformatics software and the testing platform. In addition, using an NGS platform for panel testing versus whole exome/genome testing determines the amount of surface area on the platform that is available for each region of interest. As a result, in a panel setting, where there are smaller regions of interest, a targeted capture approach provides sufficient surface area to capture reads from all available regions of this specific target. In contrast, whole exome/genome sequences require the capture of more regions of interest, limiting the area available on the platform for reads of each target. This can mean that coverage for a particular region would be better represented in a targeted panel than a whole exome/genome test.

Another limitation to NGS testing is the potential for incidental findings. An incidental finding is a variant identified in gene that is unrelated to the original reason for testing, yet potentially medically significant. For example, whole exome sequencing might be done for an individual because of a personal history of heart defects, and a pathogenic mutation is identified in a gene associated with colon cancer. The likelihood of identifying an incidental finding increases with the number of target regions available on the testing

platform; a whole exome/genome test will yield more potential incidental findings than a panel. To prepare the individuals tested, laboratories using this testing approach provide a statement on how they handle incidental findings and will provide a consent form for the individual to indicate whether he/she would/ would not like to know if an incidental finding was identified. The American College of Medical Genetics and Genomics (ACMG) has issued a guideline regarding the disclosure of incidental findings. In summary, ACMG suggests disclosure of pathogenic mutations in genes with a direct association with a known clinical condition that also has a medical surveillance, management, treatment, or cure available. The guideline then provides a list of suggested genes that meet these criteria; however, it is left up to the individual testing laboratory whether they would like to adhere to this recommendation; some have chosen to expand the list to additional genes.

Lastly, as NGS testing has been an emerging clinical technology, many clinicians and certifying bodies require or suggest that any results identified via NGS be clinically confirmed using an orthogonal technology. Currently, most laboratories confirm variants identified via NGS by Sanger sequencing.

## PRACTICAL EXAMPLES

### Somatic: BCR-ABL gene fusion.

The Philadelphia chromosome is a reciprocal translocation involving chromosomes 9 and 22 that is commonly identified in chronic myelogenous leukemia (CML). The break points of the translocation create a fusion of two genes: ABL1 on chromosome 9 and BCR on chromosome 22. The fusion gene encodes a tyrosine kinase signaling protein that leads to uncontrollable cell division. Approximately 95% of individuals with a clinical diagnosis of CML have this chromosome anomaly, enabling this to be a sensitive

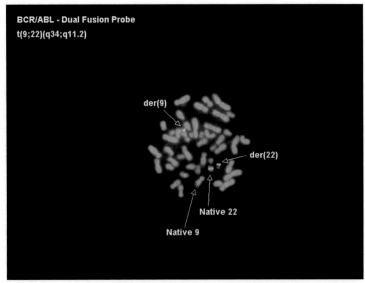

FIG. 5.9 Fluorescence in situ hybridization (FISH) probe analysis for BCR/ABL fusion probe. (Courtesy of Dr. Fady Mikhail, MD, PhD, FACMG. University of Alabama at Birmingham Cytogenetics Laboratory.)

test for clinical confirmation.[9] Identification of this translocation, however, is not specific, as it can also be found at lower detection rates in individuals with a diagnosis of acute lymphoblastic leukemia as well as acute myelogenous leukemia.

There are benefits in therapy when an individual is identified to have the BCR-ABL translocation. In the 1990s, the drug imatinib mesylate was developed as a tyrosine kinase inhibitor able to significantly limit the growth of tumor cells with the translocation. Since this time additional therapeutic agents have been created, such as dasatinib and nilotinib, with a similar mechanism of action.

### Possible testing strategy
To test for this gene fusion, live cells can be submitted for culture and karyotyping. This will detect the Philadelphia chromosome and potentially other chromosomal abnormalities (Fig. 5.10). Alternatively, FISH analysis can be performed if a faster turnaround is needed, with the fusion gene identified by labeling the ABL and BCR probes with different colors (Fig. 5.9).

### Germline: Klinefelter syndrome
Klinefelter syndrome is a sex chromosome aneuploidy that affects 1 in every 1000 newborn males. Klinefelter syndrome presents with a spectrum of phenotypes; in

fact, it is suspected that this syndrome is underdiagnosed given how mild the phenotype may be.

The most common findings in this condition are caused by low testosterone production:
- small testes
- delayed or absent puberty
- cryptorchidism
- hypospadias
- micropenis
- infertility
- gynecomastia
- reduced or absent facial and body hair

Men with Klinefelter syndrome have at least one extra X chromosome. Instead of a typical 46,XY karyotype, a male with Klinefelter may present as 47,XXY, 48,XXXY, or even more copies of the X chromosome. A karyotype analysis is the simplest way to make this diagnosis.

Men with Klinefelter syndrome are also at an increased risk for some cancers and are at a decreased risk for prostate cancer. The underlying cause for these increased risks has not been established. The incidence of each cancer risk using a standardized mortality ratio compared with that of general population[3] is listed in Table 5.6.

A karyotype or FISH for the sex chromosomes would likely be the first testing approach used to confirm this diagnosis. FISH analysis would also be most helpful to determine if there is also mosaicism. A microarray is another testing approach that could establish this

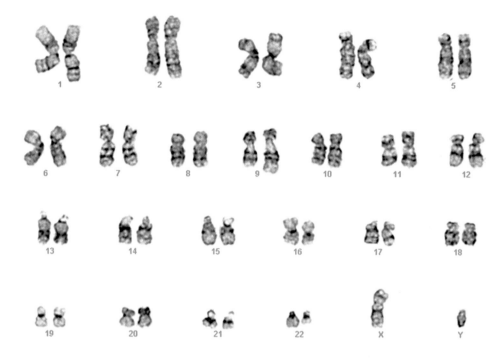

46,XY,t(9;22)(q34;q11.2)

FIG. 5.10 Karyotype analysis for chromosome 9 and 22 translocation associated with BCR/ABL fusion. (Courtesy of Dr. Fady Mikhail, MD, PhD, FACMG. University of Alabama at Birmingham Cytogenetics Laboratory.)

diagnosis; however, a microarray analysis would not be able to confidently confirm if the patient is mosaic (Fig. 5.11).

## GERMLINE TESTING: LI-FRAUMENI SYNDROME

Li-Fraumeni syndrome is a rare, autosomal dominant condition caused by mutation in the *TP53* gene. The *TP53* gene encodes a p53 protein that is unable to regulate cell growth or division. Mutations in *TP53* can be found in 50% of all tumors as somatic mutations. Individuals with Li-Fraumeni syndrome (LFS) have a greatly increased risk of developing cancer. The hallmark cancers associated with LFS are sarcomas, breast cancer, brain tumors (astrocytomas, glioblastomas, medulloblastomas, choroid plexus carcinomas), and adrenocortical carcinomas. Those with a germline mutation in the *TP53* gene are estimated to have a 50% chance of developing an LFS-related tumor by age 30 and >90% lifetime risk[10] (Table 5.7).

Although the Chompret criteria for clinical diagnosis of LFS provides a guideline for making a clinical diagnosis, identifying a causative gene mutation can be helpful in

**TABLE 5.6**
**Incidence of Cancer Rates**

| Cancer Type | Standardized Mortality Ratio |
|---|---|
| All cancers | 1.2 |
| Lung cancer | 1.5 |
| Breast cancer | 57.8 |
| Non-Hodgkin lymphoma | 3.5 |
| Prostate cancer | 0 |

recognizing asymptomatic family members who require surveillance. In addition, a few clinical predictions can be made for those with certain mutations identified (genotype-phenotype correlation). Table 5.8 lists genotype-phenotype correlations that have been identified.

## TESTING STRATEGY

To plan an appropriate testing strategy, it is important to identify the mutational spectrum seen in the condition in

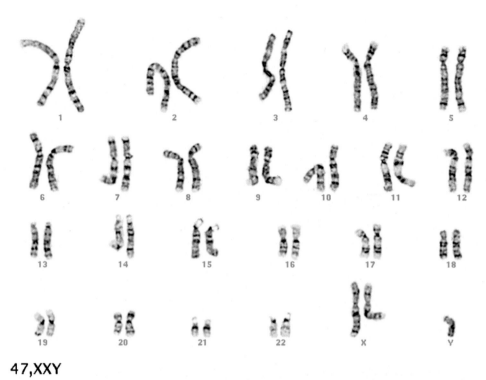

**47,XXY**

FIG. 5.11 Abnormal karyotype featuring Klinefelter syndrome. (Courtesy of Dr. Fady Mikhail, MD, PhD, FACMG. University of Alabama at Birmingham Cytogenetics Laboratory.)

**TABLE 5.7**
List of Common Tumors or Cancers Seen in Li-Fraumeni Syndrome as well as Their Lifetime Risk of Development[10]

| Location | Relative Risk (Confidence Interval 95%) |
|---|---|
| Bone | 107 (49–203) |
| Connective tissue | 61 (33–102) |
| Brain | 35 (19–60) |
| Pancreas | 7.3 (2–19) |
| Breast | 6.4 (4.3–9.3) |
| Colon | 2.8 (1–6) |
| Liver | 1.8 (2.1–64) |

**TABLE 5.8**
Genotype and Phenotype Correlations

| Genotype | Phenotype |
|---|---|
| Pathogenic missense mutations | Earlier onset of cancer |
| Total or partial gene deletions | Classic Li-Fraumeni syndrome phenotypes |
| Microdeletions involving tp53 | Lower risk for tumor formation |
| Mutations in the DNA-binding loop that contact the minor groove of DNA | Increased risk for brain tumors |
| Pathogenic mutations within the loops opposing the protein-DNA contact surface | Increased risk for adenoid cystic carcinoma |

question. 80% of families with features of LFS are found to have mutations in the TP53 gene. In addition, 95% of those with TP53 mutations are found to have variants identified via sequencing analysis and only 1% are found to have deletions/duplications in this gene. As a result, single gene Sanger sequencing would be an acceptable approach depending on a patient's clinical presentation. An adenoid cystic carcinoma tumor is more characteristic for LFS than a woman presenting with breast cancer. As a result, for one patient, a Sanger sequencing test for the TP53 gene may be the best starting point, whereas

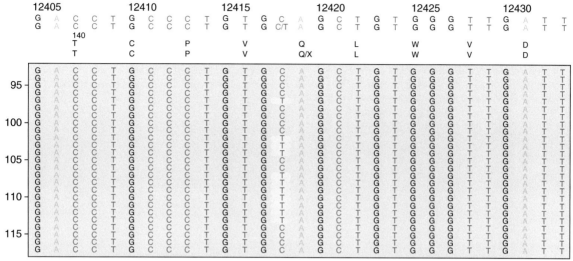

FIG. 5.12 Detection of a TP53 mutation in a patient with Li-Fraumeni syndrome. The reference sequence is shown at the top and the patient sequence below. A heterozygous C > T mutation (c.430C > T; p.Gln144X) is visible in 11 of the 25 reads shown. (Courtesy Jo Morgan and Graham Taylor, Leeds Institute of Molecular Medicine, St. James's Hospital, Leeds, UK. From Turnpenny P, Ellard S. *Emery's Elements of Medical Genetics*. Philadelphia, PA: Elsevier; 2017.)

another patient may require a multigene NGS breast cancer panel that includes the *TP53* gene. If the sequencing analysis is negative, one may consider deletion/duplication analysis as well. If the *TP53* gene is the only gene considered, MLPA analysis may be helpful for deletion/duplication analysis. If, however, several genes are under consideration for diagnosis, a microarray may be useful to look for deletions/duplications within all genes under consideration (Fig. 5.12).

## TESTING ON THE HORIZON

As technology advances and our knowledge of cancer syndromes improve, genetic testing is constantly improving. In addition, new genes and gene associations with particular cancers are also being discovered. Therefore, individuals who receive genetic testing with negative results may benefit in follow-up testing every few years as testing strategies improve.

### Cancer Screening Tests
#### Direct to consumer
Direct to consumer (DTC) tests can be ordered directly by patients, without the involvement of a health professional. While routine clinical testing options provide diagnostic results for specific genes and/or mutations, a DTC test analyzes SNPs and their statistical association with certain conditions, including cancer. Food and Drug Administration rules prevent return of clinical results based on DTC tests, unless a specific test has received approval. Nevertheless, a consumer can obtain his/her raw genotypic data, and there are services that can annotate these with potential medical conditions or risks.

#### ctDNA screening tests
Another testing approach on the horizon is the use of noninvasive cancer tests, the so-called liquid biopsy. Cell-free DNA-based testing involves NGS of circulating DNA derived from degenerating tumor cells in an individual's blood. One emerging test detects the presence of nine driver cancer genes and can provide results in 2–3 weeks.

## REFERENCES
1. Bickmore W. Karyotype analysis and chromosome banding. *eLS.* 2001:1–5.
2. Hasle H, Clemmensen IH, Mikkelsen M. Risks of leukaemia and solid tumors in individuals with Down's syndrome. *Lancet.* 2000;355(9199):165–169.
3. Swerdlow A, Shoemaker M, Higgins C, et al. Cancer incidence and mortality in men with Klinefelter syndrome: a cohort study. *J Natl Cancer Inst.* 2005;97(16):1204–1210.
4. Schneider K. *Counseling about Cancer: Strategies for Genetic Counselors.* 3rd ed. Hoboken, New Jersey: John Wiley & Sons Inc; 2012.

5. Bumgarner R. DNA microarrays: types, applications, and their future use. *Curr Protoc Mol Biol.* 2013;0 22(22.1). http://dx.doi.org/10.1002/0471142727.mb2201s101.

6. Miller D, Adam M, Aradhya S, et al. Consensus statement: chromosomal microarray is a first-tier clinical diagnostic test for individuals with developmental disabilities or congenital anomalies. *Am J Hum Genet.* 2010;86:749–764.

7. Van Veghel-Plandsoen M, Wouters C, Kromosoteo J, et al. Multiplex ligation-depending probe amplification is not suitable for detection of low-grade mosaicism. *Eur J Hum Genet.* 2011;19(9):1009–1012.

8. Hui P. Next generation sequencing: chemistry, technology and applications. *Top Curr Chem.* 2012. http://dx.doi.org/10.1007/128_2012_329.

9. Melo JV. BCR-ABL gene variants. *Baillieres Clin Haematol.* 1997;10(2):203–222.

10. Schneider K, Zelley K, Nichols KE, et al. Li-Fraumeni Syndrome. www.ncbi.nlm.nih.gov/books/NBK1311/.

# CHAPTER 6

# Genetic Syndromes With an Associated Cancer Risk

J. AUSTIN HAMM, MD

## INTRODUCTION

Children comprise a large portion of the patients who undergo evaluation by a medical geneticist. Common referral indications include congenital malformations and other unusual physical examination findings, disorders of growth and development, and inborn disorders of metabolism (IDM).[1] Many children with genetic disorders have an increased risk of specific cancers, which are characteristic of the respective genetic disorder. However, cancer is rarely the presenting sign at the initial evaluation by a medical geneticist, and these children may initially be referred to subspecialists without experience in the broader implications of that genetic syndrome, including the risk of malignancy.

The most important role for the medical geneticist in the care of children with genetic syndromes with a predisposition to cancer is to establish the correct diagnosis. With regard to cancer care, establishing the underlying genetic diagnosis is important for several reasons. First, making the correct genetic diagnosis enables appropriate surveillance for the specific malignancies associated with a given condition. For example, although both neurofibromatosis type 1 (NF1) and tuberous sclerosis complex (TSC) are genodermatoses associated with malignancies of the central nervous system, differentiating these two conditions directs clinicians to additionally monitor for either the development of malignant peripheral nerve sheath tumors (MPNSTs) in the case of NF1 or complications of usually benign angiomyolipomas in TSC. Additionally, the correct diagnosis gives patients and clinicians insight into the overall prognosis of the disorder, helps guide management, allows for adequate recurrence risk counseling, and directs families to access the appropriate support groups.

Diagnostic genetic testing may be relatively narrow when based on specific findings in the medical history or examination, such as in the case of fluorescent in situ hybridization testing or single-gene sequencing. These modalities are most useful when there is a high suspicion for specific genetic condition. However, first-line testing is usually more broad because patients often present with nonspecific symptoms, such as cognitive impairment, or because findings on physical examination do not suggest a specific diagnosis. Examples of broader testing include multigene sequencing panels, array comparative genomic hybridization (aCGH), or whole exome sequencing (WES). Additionally, widespread clinical application of whole genome sequencing is also on the horizon. As usage of genomic testing increases, the incidental detection of unsuspected genetic abnormalities is likely to increase, including abnormalities related to cancer predisposition. Furthermore, as discussed below, germline genetic abnormalities are increasingly being identified incidentally in the course of genetic testing for other indications.

Guidelines exist for the surveillance of many genetic syndromes associated with cancer predisposition. Some of these guidelines are cited within this chapter and within the next chapter, Chapter 7, Cancer Syndromes That Present in Childhood. The medical geneticist can work with the patient's other medical providers to help implement the appropriate imaging and laboratory studies. The geneticist is most helpful to the medical team when the clinical relevance of genetic findings is unclear or when the risk for cancer extends to other family members. Additionally, the geneticist will be well positioned to help translate genetic findings into clinical practice as both tumor and germline sequencing become a more routine component of pediatric cancer care.[2]

In this chapter, we will highlight several widely-recognized genetic syndromes with symptoms that present in childhood and and are associated with an increased risk of cancer. These conditions typically present for genetic evaluation for other indications, prior to developing cancer, and are therefore not considered "cancer syndromes." These syndromes are grouped by common presenting features, although there is substantial overlap among these categories.

## DYSMORPHIC FEATURES AND MULTIPLE CONGENITAL ANOMALIES

Pediatricians widely recognize the utility of a medical genetics evaluation for children with malformation syndromes. The myriad patterns of malformations can be overwhelming to both providers and families. Though medical and surgical treatment take precedence, and the focus of a genetic evaluation in such instances is often on arriving at diagnosis so as to offer a sense of closure, practitioners should not lose sight of the long term management of these conditions, including the risk of cancer.

## Trisomy 21

Trisomy 21, commonly referred to as Down syndrome, is caused by an additional copy of the 21st chromosome that typically results from a nondisjunction event during gametogenesis. Trisomy 21 is a prototypical genetic condition in which characteristic facial features (Fig. 6.1), a distinctive constellation of malformations, and cognitive impairment coalesce in a singular disorder. Medical difficulties associated with Down syndrome include hearing and vision problems, sleep apnea, otitis media, and congenital heart disease. For a detailed list of medical

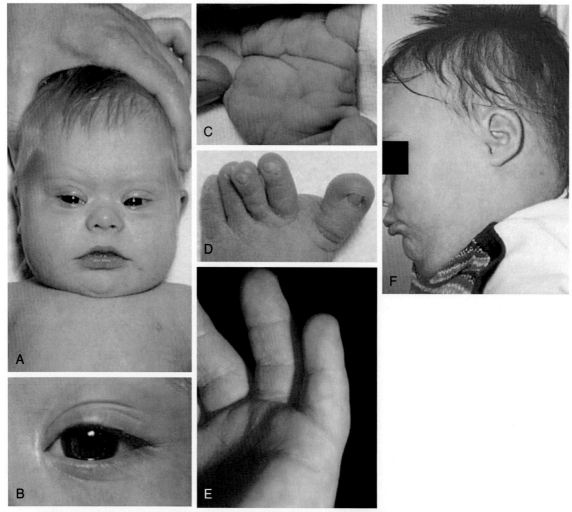

FIG. 6.1 Down syndrome. (From Ferri F. *Ferri's Color Atlas and Text of Clinical Medicine*, 2nd ed. Philadelphia, PA: Elsevier; 2009.) Clinical photographs of several minor anomalies associated with Down Syndrome. **(A)**. Characteristic facial features with upward-slanting palpebral fissures, epicanthal folds, and flat nasal bridge. **(B)**. Brushfield spots of the iris. **(C)**. Transverse palmar crease. **(D)**. Widely-spaced first and second toes. **(E)**. Short fifth finger. **(F)**. Small ears and flat occiput.

problems common in Down syndrome, see Table 6 in Bull,[4] referenced at the end of the chapter. Down syndrome is easily diagnosed with routine cytogenetic studies. This condition is among the most common genetic disorders, with an incidence of roughly 1:700 live births[3] in the United States. In addition to congenital malformations, patients with trisomy 21 are at risk for a host of other medical conditions over the course of their lifetimes, ranging from autoimmune disorder to depression and, in the context of this book, leukemias.[4]

Children with trisomy 21 have a 10- to 50-fold increased risk for leukemias compared with unaffected children,[5] and the risk of acute myeloid leukemia (AML) is especially high compared with their peers. Transient myelodysplastic disease (TMD) may occur in the newborn period of up to 5%–10% of newborns with trisomy 21,[6,7] and as many as 16%–25% of these affected children go on to develop AML.[7,8] Clinically, TMD ranges from asymptomatic mild leukocytosis to multiorgan disease, most often affecting the liver, spleen, and skin. Pathogenic variants in the *GATA1* gene, which encodes a key transcription factor that regulates hematopoiesis, can be observed in multiple hematologic disorders but are a key diagnostic feature in trisomy 21 leukemias, specifically variants in exon 2. The presence of peripheral blasts with characteristic flow cytometry coupled with detection of *GATA1* variants aid in the laboratory diagnosis of TMD. Although TMD generally self-resolves in the first months of infancy in the trisomy 21 population, complications of the disease cause death in roughly 20% of cases.[9] Liver failure, hydrops, and cardiopulmonary disease are associated with increased mortality.

Trisomy 21 is the most common condition predisposing to the development of AML in childhood. Onset typically occurs prior to 4 years of age and is often preceded by TMD or myelodysplasia with chronic cytopenias, especially isolated thrombocytopenia. Trisomy 21–associated AML (also known as Down syndrome–associated megakaryocytic leukemia or DS-AMKL) differs from other cases of AML in several ways, including an early age of onset, the presence of megakaryoblasts, and the lack of the prognostic cytogenetic rearrangements that are commonly seen in non–DS-AMKL. As in TMD, somatic pathogenic *GATA1* variants are present in almost all cases of DS-AMKL. Patients with TMD who go on to develop DS-AMKL have identical *GATA1* variants, which suggests that DS-AMKL develops from surviving monoclonal or oligoclonal TMD blasts. Prognosis for DS-AMKL is excellent compared with other forms of childhood-onset AML, with cure rates upward of 80% with intensive chemotherapy regimens.[10]

Patients with trisomy 21 are also at increased risk of lymphoid leukemias. Although acute lymphoblastic leukemia (ALL) in trisomy 21 does not represent a distirct clinical entity, such as DS-AMKL, it does vary from cases of ALL that are not associated with trisomy 21. Trisomy 21 patients are less likely to have the common t(12;21)(p13;q22) (Lanza, 1997) or t(1;19)(q23;p13) rearrangements,[11] are less likely to have T-cell or mature B-cell ALL subtypes, and have more severe symptoms related to chemotherapy toxicity compared with ALL patients without trisomy 21. Overall survival rates of patients with trisomy 21 with ALL lag behind the survival rate of those with ALL who are not affected with trisomy 21, although some studies suggest overall survival of these two groups is comparable when controlled for biologic features of the cancers.[12]

Although the increased risk for leukemias persists until the fourth decade of life, individuals with trisomy 21 are at a lower risk for solid tumor cancers, particularly in middle and late adulthood. A 2016 study found that the risk of lung, breast, and cervical cancer is significantly reduced, and of solid tumors, only testicular cancer posed an increased risk to individuals with trisomy 21.[13] Although some environmental exposures, such as decreased tobacco use and decreased sexual activity, may contribute to this apparent protective effect, these are unlikely to explain the entirety of the risk reduction, especially because the trisomy 21 population has an increase in some other risk factors for cancer, such as accelerated aging, obesity, and nulliparity. The combination of increased risk of leukemia and decreased risk of solid tumors makes trisomy 21 a useful model for studying carcinogenesis.

### Wilms Tumor, Aniridia, Genitourinary Malformations, Mental Retardation Syndrome

WAGR (Wilms tumor, aniridia, genitourinary malformations, mental retardation) is a genetic syndrome characterized by congenital anomalies, including aniridia and genitourinary malformations, intellectual disability, and increased risk of Wilms tumor (WT) in childhood. In addition to aniridia (Fig. 6.2), other common pathologic eye findings that can be seen include cataracts, glaucoma, and nystagmus. The most commonly observed genitourinary malformation in affected males is undescended testes, whereas females may be affected with streak gonads or uterine malformations.[14] The genetic defect responsible for WAGR is an interstitial microdeletion of the 11p13 region. Although phenotype may vary with the size of the microdeletion, deletion of *PAX6*, *WT1*, and *PRRG4* appear critical to the classical phenotype.[15,16] Deletions that extend to encompass the *BDNF*, a gene in which defects may

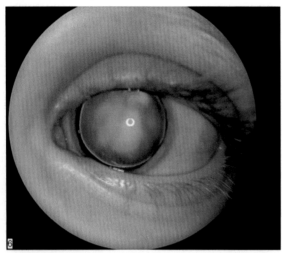

FIG. 6.2 Aniridia. (From Traboulsi EI. Aniridia. In: Levin LA, Albert DM, eds. *Ocular Disease: Mechanisms and Management*. Philadelphia, PA: Elsevier; 2017:472–477 [Chapter 61].)

result in monogenic obesity, can result in a subtype of WAGR, which is sometimes abbreviated as WAGRO syndrome for the addition of obesity.

WT is the most common renal malignancy of childhood, affecting up to 1 in 8000 children.[17] WT is thought to develop from persistent embryonal kidney cells, collections of which are known as nephrogenic rests. Germline abnormalities in *WT1*, a gene that encodes a key transcription factor that helps direct growth and differentiation of renal cells, are responsible for up to 15% of cases of WT.[18] One copy of *WT1* is lost in WAGR syndrome, and pathogenic sequence variants in *WT1* are responsible for Denys-Drash syndrome and Frasier syndrome, which are other genetic conditions associated with genitourinary malformations and an increased risk of WT.

WT often presents as an asymptomatic abdominal mass in a preschool-age child. Some children may also demonstrate fever, abdominal pain, anemia, hematuria, and/or hypertension. Onset prior to 3 years of age and/or the presence of bilateral malignancies are associated with an increased risk of germline genetic abnormalities. WT rarely occurs in adulthood.

Surgical resection is key to Wilms tumor treatment. Patients with unilateral malignancy undergo nephrectomy, whereas those with bilateral malignancy may elect to have nephron-sparing resection of the tumor. All patients are additionally treated with chemotherapy. Radiation therapy, in addition to more aggressive chemotherapy regimens, is used in instances of advanced disease. Overall survival in cases of favorable histology ranges from 86.1% (stage IV) to 98.4% (stage I); survival in cases of anaplastic histology varies from 37.5% to 82.6% depending on the stage. 10%–15% of affected patients have a relapse of WT, and with modern treatment regimens, survival in relapse cases is roughly 50%–60%.[18]

Patients with history of WT undergo serial chest X-rays and abdominal ultrasounds for evidence of disease recurrence. Surveillance in patients with a genetic predisposition to WT who have not yet developed the disease should include abdominal ultrasounds every 3 months. This includes patients with WAGR and other disorders associated with *WT1* defects, as well as disorders associated with hemihypertrophy, such as Beckwith-Wiedemann syndrome (BWS).

As in other disorders affecting the development of the genitals, patients with WAGR syndrome are at an increased risk of gonadoblastoma. In some of the early reports of WAGR cases, the "G" referred to gonadoblastoma, rather than genitourinary malformations, because of the association with this disease, and although WT is a much more common malignancy in children with WAGR, these patients should also be monitored for gonadoblastoma. In females with streak gonads due to WAGR, surveillance for development of gonadoblastoma using MRI of the pelvis is appropriate.

## ABNORMALITIES OF GROWTH

Abnormal patterns of growth, including failure to thrive, short stature, overgrowth, and body asymmetry, are common causes of referral to a genetic specialist. The workup for these findings can be complex and includes obtaining detailed social, dietary, developmental, and family histories. In addition to the primary care provider, geneticists often work in conjunction with endocrinologists, gastroenterologists, and other specialists when evaluating affected patients. Although the majority of cases are due to environmental factors or constitutional genetic influences, some instances of abnormal growth are due to discrete genetic abnormalities, and a significant subset of these disorders are associated with cancer predisposition.

### Fanconi Anemia

Fanconi anemia (FA) is a heterogeneous disorder characterized by bone marrow failure, endocrinologic abnormalities and congenital malformations. At least 15 different genes have been detected in which defects cause FA, and with the exception of the X-linked *FANCB*, the disorder is transmitted in an autosomal recessive manner. These genes encode the proteins responsible for a DNA repair mechanism that helps resolve DNA interstrand cross-links, which impair normal DNA replication. The presence of these cross-links forms the basis of chromosomal breakage analysis, which is a nongenetic method that helps make an FA diagnosis. On exposure to DNA cross-linking agents, lymphocytic chromosomes of patients with FA demonstrate increased occurrences of chromosomal breakage relative to normal controls. In cases of high clinical suspicion for FA, skin biopsy and testing of fibroblasts, rather than lymphocytes, is warranted because of the relatively high incidence of somatic mosaicism in this population.

Classically, patients with FA demonstrate short stature, increased skin pigmentation, and radial ray defects, which may manifest as hypoplasia or aplasia of the thumb. However, other findings such a microcephaly, ophthalmologic abnormalities, and genitourinary malformations may be present. Roughly a quarter of patients may have some degree of intellectual disability. About 60% of patients with FA have short stature,[19,20] which is often, but not universally, associated with endocrinopathy. Because of the clinical variability of this condition, it is an important diagnosis to exclude when evaluating a child for short stature, because other characteristic findings of FA may be absent. FA patients are at increased risk of a wide range of endocrinologic disorders, including growth hormone deficiency, hypothyroidism, and hypogonadism, among others. Biallelic pathogenic *FANCD1* variants are notably associated with earlier onset of leukemia and solid tumors, and heterozygous carriers are also at increased risk of malignancy, especially breast, ovarian, and pancreatic cancer. In the context of heterozygous variants, *FANCD1* is more often referred to as *BRCA2*, variants in which are widely recognized as causing autosomal dominant BRCA-related breast and/or ovarian cancer syndrome, previously referred to as hereditary breast and ovarian cancer.

Although as many as 40% of FA patients do not demonstrate significant outward signs of the disorder,[21] up to 90% will have some degree of bone marrow failure. Roughly 50% of these patients will develop myelodysplastic syndrome or AML. Additionally, 75% of FA patients will develop solid tumors,[22] including liver adenomas and hepatomas as well as malignancies of the aerodigestive and gynecologic tracts. Notably, as many as 25% of patients diagnosed with FA develop a cancer prior to being diagnosed.[23]

Hematopoietic stem cell transplant (HSCT) remains the mainstay of treatment for bone marrow failure associated with FA. However, due to faulty DNA

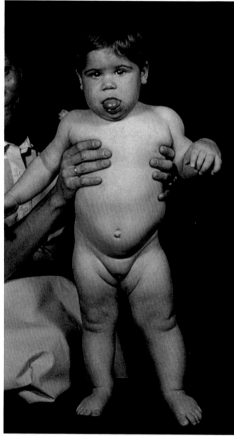

FIG. 6.3 A young child with Beckwith–Wiedemann syndrome. Note the macroglossia and left leg hemihyperplasia. (From *Zitelli and Davis Atlas of Pediatric Physical Diagnosis*. 6th ed. Philadelphia, PA: Elsevier; 2012.)

repair, patients with FA have historically suffered higher degrees of toxicity related to the chemotherapy and radiation treatments that are necessary for HSCT. Although recent developments of lower-dose treatment regimens have mitigated this increased susceptibility toxicity, FA patients remain at an increased risk of secondary cancers and require ongoing surveillance.

### Beckwith-Wiedemann Syndrome

BWS is caused by abnormalities of the imprinting cluster located at 11p15 and is characterized by somatic overgrowth, characteristic facial features, visceromegaly with predisposition to development of omphalocele, and a predisposition to embryonal tumors. In the newborn period, patients with BWS may have hypoglycemia or polycythemia and are at risk of a respiratory compromise due to airway obstruction from macroglossia (Fig. 6.3).

Growth of the oral cavity usually causes macroglossia to become less prominent with age, but severe cases may necessitate partial glossectomy in infancy. Overgrowth begins prenatally and slows during childhood, with the final adult height falling within normal limits.

BWS has a very heterogeneous and complex genetic etiology, as its possible causes include copy number variants (CNVs), sequence variants, or imprinting errors. Imprinting disorders involve epigenetic modifications to nuclear DNA, and clinical symptoms vary based on the parent of origin. DNA methylation at imprinting centers is a common mechanism of epigenetic regulation, and these epigenetic marks are erased from one generation to the next. Although the 11p15 imprinted centers contain multiple genes that regulate growth, it is instructive to consider one of these genes, *IGF2*, which encodes insulin-like growth factor 2, as it relates to the pathogenesis of BWS. *IGF2* is expressed from the paternal allele, and genetic changes, such as paternal uniparental disomy of chr11, duplication of the paternal 11p15 region, or certain primary methylation errors, cause increased expression of *IGF2*, which contributes to the symptoms of BWS. Notably, different genetic defects involving the 11p15 region, including maternal uniparental disomy of chr11, cause Russell-Silver syndrome, a genetic disorder whose hallmark feature is short stature.

The recurrence risk of BWS varies based on the genetic cause of the disorder, and BWS is not heritable in most cases. In up to 15% of cases, BWS is transmitted due to CNVs or gene sequence variants in an autosomal dominant fashion, although symptoms vary according to the parent of origin. Methylation defects are not heritable, and monozygotic twins discordant for BWS have been observed to have primary methylation defects. Although the overall incidence remains low, assisted reproductive technologies have been associated with an increased risk of syndromes caused by methylation defects, including BWS.

Individuals with BWS are at increased risk for developing embryonal tumors, such as hepatoblastoma, WT, and adrenocortical carcinoma, among others. The overall risk of tumor development in patients with BWS has been estimated at 8.8%,[24] with the majority of tumors forming prior to 8 years of age. Serial serum α-fetoprotein levels and renal ultrasound are conducted every 3 months until age 8 as tumor surveillance. BWS patients with hemihypertrophy appear to be at the highest risk of malignancy, and the American College of Medical Genetics recommends the same screening protocol for any patient with hemihypertrophy, even if a diagnosis of BWS is not suspected or confirmed.[25]

## DERMATOLOGIC ABNORMALITIES

Patients with genetic disorders display a diverse array of dermatologic abnormalities that may be associated with anomalies of nearby tissues, such as nail and hair, or with defects of other tissues of ectodermal origin, such as nerves and teeth. Some of these diseases also cause predisposition to cancer. In contrast to many cancer predisposition syndromes, dermal findings are often readily apparent to the patient, the family, and medical providers, offering an opportunity to make the correct diagnosis in a timely fashion with implementation of cancer surveillance as indicated.

### Neurofibromatosis[26]

With an incidence of up to 1 in 3000,[27] NF is among the most common genetic disorders. The most common form of this disease is NF type 1 and is caused by defects in the *NF1* gene, which encodes a tumor suppressor that is highly expressed in oligodendrocytes and Schwann cells. Key diagnostic features of NF type 1 are neurofibromas, café-au-lait spots, axillary and inguinal freckling, pseudoarthrosis, Lisch nodules, and optic gliomas (Fig. 6.4). Molecular testing of *NF1* is widely available, although the physical features are consistent enough that the diagnosis is often made clinically.

Although neurofibromas are benign tumors, they can affect virtually any nerve of the body, and medical complications due to impingement on surrounding tissues can be significant, especially when involving large plexiform neurofibromas. In addition to peripheral tumors, NF type 1 patients are also at increased risk of central nervous system gliomas, which may be life-threatening due to their anatomic location, even if not technically malignant. The most prevalent malignancy that affects NF type1 patients is MPNST, which develops in up to 10% of patients.[28] Patients with whole gene deletions of *NF1* or who are observed to carry a high burden of clinical disease are at the highest risk.[29] MPNSTs are aggressive malignancies that arise from the multiple cell types that compose the connective tissue surrounding peripheral nerves. Surgery with wide excisional margins is the treatment of choice, and radiation is frequently used as adjuvant therapy. For MPNSTs of a limb, amputation of that extremity is frequently the treatment of choice.

Like *NF1*, the *NF2* gene is categorized as a tumor suppressor gene, but defects in this gene cause a clinically distinct disorder known as NF type 2. Although it carries a similar name, it is important to recognize that NF type 2 is clinically distinct from NF type 1. As opposed to NF type 1, in which cutaneous findings are key to the clinical diagnosis, patients with NF type 2 generally develop internal neuronal tumors, which are

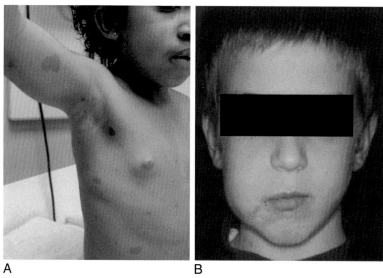

A                                            B

FIG. 6.4 Clinical findings seen in neurofibromatosis type I. **(A)** Café-au-lait macules and axillary freckling. **(B)** Facial plexiform neurofibroma. (**(A)** From Nebesio TD, Eugster EA, Current concepts in normal and abnormal puberty. *Curr Probl Pediatr Adolesc Health Care*. 2008;37(2):50–72; with permission. **(B)** From Fadda MT, Verdino G, Mustazza MC, Bartoli D, Iannetti G. Intra-parotid facial nerve multiple plexiform neurofibroma in patient with NF1. *Int J Pediatr Otorhinolaryngol*. 2008;72:553–557.)

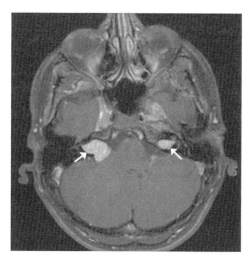

FIG. 6.5 MRI of neurofibromatosis type 2, demonstrating bilateral VIIIth nerve schwanomas (arrows). (From Mirvis SE, Kubal WS, Shanmuganathan K, et al. *Problem Solving in Emergency Radiology*. Philadelphia, PA: Elsevier; 2014.)

usually not evident on routine physical examination. Vestibular schwannoma is the tumor most commonly associated with NF type 2 (Fig. 6.5), and hearing loss and tinnitus are the most common presenting complaints of patients with this disorder. Patients with

NF type 2 often develop vestibular schwannomas in early adulthood, and they are frequently bilateral. Other associated tumors are meningiomas, gliomas, and other schwannomas. Although these tumors are usually benign, their anatomic position can cause significant morbidity or mortality. NF type 2 is generally diagnosed in adulthood, but children or adolescents may come to clinical attention for cutaneous schwannomas or eye problems, such as cataracts or retinal hamartomas, which are also features of this disorder.

## Xeroderma Pigmentosum

Xeroderma pigmentosum (XP) is caused by genetic defects in any one of many genes that encode proteins of the DNA repair system responsible for excising and mending DNA damaged by the formation of pyrimidine dimers. Pyrimidine dimers form during a photochemical reaction usually prompted by exposure to UV light in which covalent bonds form within neighboring bases of the same DNA strand. This reaction disrupts the normal hydrogen bonding between bases on opposite strands and distorts DNA structure. Additionally, the cell sometimes resolves this abnormality by inducing a point mutation at the affected site, which can be maladaptive.

Nucleotide excision repair is the process by which the cell effectively corrects pyrimidine dimers, and defects in this repair system result in the clinical phenotype of XP. XP is characterized by photosensitivity and many dermatologic abnormalities, including a marked susceptibility to skin cancers. The incidence of XP is roughly 1:1,000,000 in western countries,[30] although incidence in Japan has been estimated to be as high as 1:22,000.[31] The disorder is transmitted in an autosomal recessive manner.

Dermatologic findings in XP include irregular pigmentation and diffuse freckling, cutaneous telangiectasias, generalized atrophy and xerosis of skin, and a history of sunburns with minimal light exposure (Fig. 6.6). The majority of affected patients display cutaneous symptoms by the age of 3 years, and many develop skin cancer within the first decade of life. Additionally, UV exposure of ocular structures leads to photophobia, conjunctivitis, and keratitis. Roughly a quarter of XP patients also suffer from neurologic abnormalities, which range from mild to severe. Severely affected patients may demonstrate progressive neurologic disease with cognitive impairment, microcephaly, hearing loss, spasticity, and/or epilepsy. Management of XP requires prompt diagnosis and focuses mainly on the prevention of symptoms by attempting to minimize UV exposure and engaging in rigorous tumor surveillance. Retinoids or immunomodulating medications have been used in some patients for tumor prevention. Both dermatologic and ophthalmologic symptoms frequently require surgical intervention.

Basal cell carcinomas and squamous cell carcinomas are the most common types of malignancy in XP and are first observed in childhood and adolescence, which precedes the typical occurrence of these tumors in unaffected patients by over 50 years. Melanomas are also frequent and often develop in late adolescence and early adulthood. Compared with unaffected individuals, the risk of nonmelanoma skin cancer in individuals with XP is increased 10,000-fold and the risk of melanoma is increased 2000-fold.[32] Counterintuitively, patients without the history of susceptibility to sunburns are more likely to develop skin cancers. This may be explained by behavioral modification in response to frequent burns. Additionally, patients with XP are at an increased risk of oral cancers and a variety of internal cancers, which occur 10–20 times more often in these patients compared with the general population.[33] XP is associated with early mortality, with over half of patients dying before 40 years of age. Skin cancer is the most common cause of death, although nearly a third of patients die from complications of neurologic disease. Internal cancers are also a significant cause of mortality in XP patients.

## INBORN DISORDERS OF METABOLISM

IDM are a diverse group of rare diseases in which genetic abnormalities cause disruption of biochemical pathways. Although management of these conditions is often focused on specialized diets or emergent treatment during potentially life-threatening episodes of metabolic decompensation, cancer surveillance is also necessary in some of these disorders. For example, patients with Gaucher disease, a lysosomal storage disorder caused by deficiency of glucocerebrosidase and characterized by hepatosplenomegaly, cytopenias, lung disease, and painful crises associated with bone disease, are at an increased risk of multiple myeloma and hematologic malignancies. These patients also appear to have an overall increased risk of cancer, with relative risk being 1.70 compared with unaffected individuals.[34] Increased risks of hepatocellular carcinoma (HCC),[35] malignant melanoma, and pancreatic cancer[36] have specifically been reported, although these associations are not as clear.

The liver is perhaps the most crucial site of metabolism in the human body, and multiple IDM are associated with HCC. As toxic metabolites accumulate because of enzymatic defects, chronic damage is done to the liver, leading to cirrhosis and/or malignancy. Hereditary hemochromatosis, Wilson disease, $\alpha_1$-antitrypsin deficiency, tyrosinemia, and multiple glycogen storage diseases are among the most recognized genetic diseases associated with an increased risk of HCC. Guidelines for surveillance of populations at risk of HCC recommend obtaining periodic liver ultrasounds and serum $\alpha$ protein levels. However, these recommendations generally apply to more common causes of cirrhosis, such as alcoholism or infectious hepatitis, and guidelines for HCC screening in patients with inborn errors of metabolism are less standardized.

## INCIDENTAL DETECTION OF GENETIC CANCER PREDISPOSITION

Although many genetic syndromes are associated with increased cancer risk, cancer predisposition is rarely the primary referral indication for children who visit a medical geneticist. If a patient is suspected of having a genetic condition that has an attendant risk of malignancy, the family may be counseled about this risk on confirmation of the diagnosis or when testing for the disorder is being sent. However, with the increased use of advanced clinical genetics testing methods, such as aCGH and WES, genetic cancer predisposition may be detected incidentally without regard to a patient's presenting symptoms.

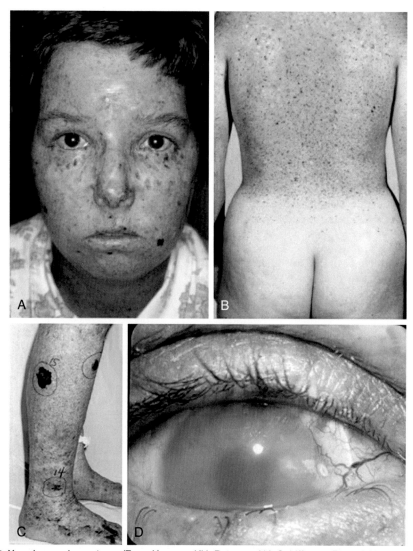

FIG. 6.6 Xeroderma pigmentosa. (From Kraemer KH, Patronas NJ, Schiffmann R, et al. Xeroderma pigmentosum, trichothiodystrophy and Cockayne syndrome: a complex genotype-phenotype relationship. *Neuroscience*. April 14, 2007;145(4):1388–1396. Epub 2007 Feb 1.) Skin and eye involvement in XP.
**(A)** Poikilodermatous changes of face with areas of increased freckle-like pigmentation, areas of decreased pigment and atrophy. The lips show cheilitis and there is absence of eye lashes on both lower lids.
**(B)** Back demonstrating similar dermatologic changes with a sharp cutoff at her sun-protected buttocks.
**(C)** Right calf with multiple large pigmented lesions. Lesion 15 was a large melanoma that measured 0.55 mm in depth when excised. **(D)** Eye demonstrating clouding of the cornea, prominent vascular growth on the conjunctiva approaching the limbus and loss of lashes on the lower lid.

Additionally, genetic test results may report abnormalities of genes associated with cancer predisposition that are of uncertain clinical significance, which may raise difficult questions for providers and family that is regarding the need for cancer surveillance. For

example, up to 1.6% of aCGH results from a medical genetics clinic may demonstrate a copy number variation of a known cancer predisposition gene, although only 0.34% of such results are clearly cancer predisposing. Among children with an abnormal aCGH result, those values increase to 5.4% and 1.2%, respectively.[37] Although cancer risk associated with copy number variations of some genes, such as a deletion of *RB1*, is well understood, the absolute risk of cancer in the instance of structural genetic abnormalities is frequently unknown.

Furthermore, the use of WES in diverse clinical contexts increases the likelihood of detecting pathogenic variants incidentally. Up to 4.6% of patients who undergo WES have been found to harbor medically actionable incidental findings.[38] In 2013, the American College of Medical Genetics issued a list of 56 genes for which they recommended reporting incidentally detected pathogenic variants, even if the results were apparently unrelated to the patient's presenting symptoms.[39] Many of the genes on this list are associated with cancer predisposition syndromes. In the past, pediatric cancers were often dismissed as sporadic, but recent evidence suggests that 8.5%–10% of pediatric cancer cases may be associated with germline genetic sequence abnormalities in known cancer predisposition genes, regardless of family history.[40,41] Recognition of genetic risk factors for cancer development will continue to increase as the use of WES and whole genome sequencing expands into routine clinical practice.

## REFERENCES

1. Pletcher BA, Toriello HV, Noblin SJ, et al. Indications for genetic referral: a guide for healthcare providers. *Genet Med.* 2007;9(6):385–389. http://dx.doi.org/10.1097/GIM.0b013e318064e70c.
2. Mody RJ, Wu Y-M, Lonigro RJ, et al. Integrative clinical sequencing in the management of refractory or relapsed cancer in youth. *JAMA.* 2015;314(9):913–925. http://dx.doi.org/10.1001/jama.2015.10080.
3. Parker SE, Mai CT, Canfield MA, et al. Updated national birth prevalence estimates for selected birth defects in the United States, 2004-2006. *Birth Defects Res A Clin Mol Teratol.* 2010;88(12):1008–1016. http://dx.doi.org/10.1002/bdra.20735.
4. Bull MJ. Health supervision for children with Down syndrome. *Pediatrics.* 2011;128(2):393–406. http://dx.doi.org/10.1542/peds.2011-1605.
5. Nižetić D, Groet J. Tumorigenesis in Down's syndrome: big lessons from a small chromosome. *Nat Rev Cancer.* 2012;12(10):721–732. http://dx.doi.org/10.1038/nrc3355.
6. Malinge S, Izraeli S, Crispino JD. Insights into the manifestations, outcomes, and mechanisms of leukemogenesis in down syndrome. *Blood.* 2009;113(12):2619–2628. http://dx.doi.org/10.1182/blood-2008-11-163501.
7. Zipursky A, Brown E, Christensen H, Sutherland R, Doyle J. Leukemia and/or myeloproliferative syndrome in neonates with Down syndrome. *Semin Perinatol.* 1997;21:97–101. http://dx.doi.org/10.1016/S0146-0005(97)80025-0.

8. Gamis AS, Alonzo TA, Gerbing RB, et al. Natural history of transient myeloproliferative disorder clinically diagnosed in Down syndrome neonates: a report from the Children's Oncology Group Study A2971. *Blood.* 2011;118(26):6752–6759. http://dx.doi.org/10.1182/blood-2011-04-350017.
9. Muramatsu H, Kato K, Watanabe N, et al. Risk factors for early death in neonates with Down syndrome and transient leukaemia. *Br J Haematol.* 2008;142(4):610–615. http://dx.doi.org/10.1111/j.1365-2141.2008.07231.x.
10. Creutzig U, Reinhardt D, Diekamp S, Dworzak M, Stary J, Zimmermann M. AML patients with Down syndrome have a high cure rate with AML-BFM therapy with reduced dose intensity. *Leukemia.* 2005;19(8):1355–1360. http://dx.doi.org/10.1038/sj.leu.2403814.
11. Pui CH, Raimondi SC, Borowitz MJ, et al. Immunophenotypes and karyotypes of leukemic cells in children with Down syndrome and acute lymphoblastic leukemia. *J Clin Oncol.* 1993;11(7):1361–1367.
12. Maloney KW, Carroll WL, Carroll AJ, et al. Down syndrome childhood acute lymphoblastic leukemia has a unique spectrum of sentinel cytogenetic lesions that influences treatment outcome: a report from the Children's Oncology Group. *Blood.* 2010;116(7):1045–1050. http://dx.doi.org/10.1182/blood-2009-07-235291.
13. Hasle H, Friedman JM, Olsen JH, Rasmussen SA. Low risk of solid tumors in persons with Down syndrome. *Genet Med.* November 2016;18:1–7. http://dx.doi.org/10.1038/gim.2016.23.
14. Wagr-Syndrome @ ghr.nlm.nih.gov.
15. Yamamoto T, Togawa M, Shimada S, Sangu N, Shimojima K, Okamoto N. Narrowing of the responsible region for severe developmental delay and autistic behaviors in WAGR syndrome down to 1.6Mb including PAX6, WT1, and PRRG4. *Am J Med Genet A.* 2014;164(3):634–638. http://dx.doi.org/10.1002/ajmg.a.36325.
16. Xu S, Han JC, Morales A, Menzie CM, Williams K, Fan YS. Characterization of 11p14-p12 deletion in WAGR syndrome by array CGH for identifying genes contributing to mental retardation and autism. *Cytogenet Genome Res.* 2008;122(2):181–187. http://dx.doi.org/10.1159/000172086.
17. Breslow N, Olshan A, Beckwith JB, Green DM. Epidemiology of Wilms tumor. *Med Pediatr Oncol.* 1993;21(3):172–181. http://dx.doi.org/10.1002/mpo.2950210305.
18. Dome J, Huff V. Wilms tumor predisposition. In: Pagon RA, Adam MP, Ardinger HH, et al., eds. *GeneReviews® [Internet].* Seattle, WA: University of Washington; 2003. 1993-2017.
19. Rose SR, Myers KC, Rutter MM, et al. Endocrine phenotype of children and adults with Fanconi anemia. *Pediatr Blood Cancer.* 2012;59(4):690–696. http://dx.doi.org/10.1002/pbc.24095.
20. Petryk A, Shankar RK, Giri N, et al. Endocrine disorders in Fanconi anemia: recommendations for screening and treatment. *J Clin Endocrinol Metab.* 2015;100(3):803–811. http://dx.doi.org/10.1210/jc.2014-4357.
21. Kee Y, D'Andrea A. Molecular pathogenesis and clinical management of Fanconi anemia. *J Clin Invest.* 2012;122(11):3799–3806. http://dx.doi.org/10.1172/JCI58321.anomalies.

22. Rosenberg PS, Greene MH, Alter BP. Cancer incidence in persons with Fanconi anemia. *Blood.* 2003;101(3):822–826. http://dx.doi.org/10.1182/blood-2002-05-1498.

23. Alter BP. Cancer in Fanconi anemia, 1927-2001. *Cancer.* 2003;97(2):425–440. http://dx.doi.org/10.1002/cncr.11046.

24. Tan TY, Amor DJ. Tumour surveillance in Beckwith-Wiedemann syndrome and hemihyperplasia: a critical review of the evidence and suggested guidelines for local practice. *J Paediatr Child Health.* 2006;42(9):486–490. http://dx.doi.org/10.1111/j.1440-1754.2006.00908.x.

25. Clericuzio CL, Martin RA. Diagnostic criteria and tumor screening for individuals with isolated hemihyperplasia. *Genet Med.* 2009;11(3):220–222. http://dx.doi.org/10.1097/GIM.0b013e31819436cf.

26. Korf B, Rubenstein A. In: Hiscock T, Brandenburg B, eds. *Neurofibromatosis: A Handbook for Patients, Families and Health Care Professionals.* 2nd ed. New York: Thieme Medical Publishers; 2011.

27. *Neurofibromatosis Type 1. Genetics Home Reference.* 2016. https://ghr.nlm.nih.gov/condition/neurofibromatosis-type-1#statistics.

28. McCaughan JA, Holloway SM, Davidson R, Lam WWK. Further evidence of the increased risk for malignant peripheral nerve sheath tumour from a Scottish cohort of patients with neurofibromatosis type 1. *J Med Genet.* 2007;44(7):463–466. http://dx.doi.org/10.1136/jmg.2006.048140.

29. Tucker T, Wolkenstein P, Revuz J, Zeller J, Friedman JM. Association between benign and malignant peripheral nerve sheath tumors in NF1. *Neurology.* 2005;65(2):205–211. http://dx.doi.org/10.1212/01.wnl.0000168830.79997.13.

30. Kleijer WJ, Laugel V, Berneburg M, et al. Incidence of DNA repair deficiency disorders in western Europe: xeroderma pigmentosum, Cockayne syndrome and trichothiodystrophy. *DNA Repair (Amst).* 2008;7(5):744–750. http://dx.doi.org/10.1016/j.dnarep.2008.01.014.

31. Hirai Y, Kodama Y, Moriwaki SI, et al. Heterozygous individuals bearing a founder mutation in the XPA DNA repair gene comprise nearly 1% of the Japanese population. *Mutat Res.* 2006;601(1–2):171–178. http://dx.doi.org/10.1016/j.mrfmmm.2006.06.010.

32. Bradford PT, Goldstein AM, Tamura D, et al. Cancer and neurologic degeneration in xeroderma pigmentosum: long term follow-up characterises the role of DNA repair. *J Med Genet.* 2011;48(3):168–176. http://dx.doi.org/10.1136/jmg.2010.083022.

33. Kraemer K, DiGiovanna J. Xeroderma pigmentosum. In: *GeneReviews.* 2016. https://www.ncbi.nlm.nih.gov/books/NBK1397/.

34. Arends M, Van Dussen L, Biegstraaten M, Hollak CEM. Malignancies and monoclonal gammopathy in Gaucher disease; a systematic review of the literature. *Br J Haematol.* 2013;161(6):832–842. http://dx.doi.org/10.1111/bjh.12335.

35. de Fost M, Vom Dahl S, Weverling GJ, et al. Increased incidence of cancer in adult Gaucher disease in Western Europe. *Blood Cells Mol Dis.* 2006;36(1):53–58. http://dx.doi.org/10.1016/j.bcmd.2005.08.004.

36. Landgren O, Turesson I, Gridley G, Caporaso NE. Risk of malignant disease among 1525 adult male US Veterans with Gaucher disease. *Arch Intern Med.* 2007;167(11):1189–1194. http://dx.doi.org/10.1001/archinte.167.11.1189.

37. Hamm JA, Mikhail FM, Hollenbeck D, Farmer M, Robin NH. Incidental detection of cancer predisposition gene copy number variations by array comparative genomic hybridization. *J Pediatr.* 2014;165(5). http://dx.doi.org/10.1016/j.jpeds.2014.07.042. 1057–1059.e4.

38. Yang Y, Muzny DM, Xia F, et al. Molecular findings among patients referred for clinical whole-exome sequencing. *JAMA.* 2014;312(18):1870. http://dx.doi.org/10.1001/jama.2014.14601.

39. Green RC, Berg JS, Grody WW, et al. ACMG recommendations for reporting of incidental findings in clinical exome and genome sequencing. *Genet Med.* 2013;15(7):565–574. http://dx.doi.org/10.1038/gim.2013.73.

40. Zhang J, Walsh MF, Wu G, et al. Germline mutations in predisposition genes in pediatric cancer. *N Engl J Med.* 2015;373(24):2336–2346. http://dx.doi.org/10.1056/NEJMoa1508054.

41. Parsons DW, Roy A, Yang Y, et al. Diagnostic yield of clinical tumor and germline whole-exome sequencing for children with solid tumors. *JAMA Oncol.* 2016;1200:1–9. http://dx.doi.org/10.1001/jamaoncol.2015.5699.

42. Lanza C, Volpe G, Basso G, Gottardi E, Perfetto F, Cilli V, Spinelli M, Ricotti E, Guerrasio A, Madon E, Saglio G. The common TEL/AML1 rearrangement does not represent a frequent event in acute lymphoblastic leukaemia occuring in children with Down syndrome. *Leukemia.* 1997; 11(6):820–821.

# CHAPTER 7

# Cancer Syndromes That Present in Childhood

KATIE FARMER, MS, CGC

## INTRODUCTION

The following chapter summarizes 15 different hereditary cancer predisposition syndromes that are associated with increased risk of benign and malignant tumors in the pediatric patient (infancy to late adolescence). This is not an exhaustive list but includes the main conditions that might be encountered in pediatric cancer genetics practice. Syndromes are organized alphabetically for ease of identification when using this text as a reference. The main clinical features, cancer risks, molecular causes, testing options, and surveillance guidelines are described and/or referenced. Please be aware that the field of pediatric hereditary cancer syndromes is quickly evolving and updated cancer risk information and management/surveillance guidelines will be available in the future.

## CONSTITUTIONAL MISMATCH REPAIR DEFICIENCY

Constitutional mismatch repair deficiency (CMMRD, also sometimes referred to as biallelic MMRD) is a childhood-onset hereditary cancer syndrome that results in significant increased risks for gastrointestinal (GI) cancers, brain tumors, and hematologic malignancies. Other cancer types have been reported at lower frequencies, and nonmalignant features, such as adenomatous polyps and café au lait macules, are very common.[1] It is an autosomal recessive condition, meaning it occurs when a child has homozygous or compound heterozygous mutations in both alleles (copies) of one of the four mismatch repair genes: *MLH1*, *MSH2*, *MSH6*, and *PMS2*. Alternatively, a child may have this condition because of a mutation in both *MSH2* and *EPCAM*, neighboring genes. Consanguinity is a common finding for the parents of affected children. Individuals who are heterozygous for an MMR gene mutation have the common hereditary cancer syndrome known as Lynch syndrome.[2]

The European Consortium "Care for CMMR-D" has developed scoring criteria for when to consider testing a child for CMMRD.[3]

Because of CMMRD being a relatively newly described and rare condition, detailed data for lifetime cancer risks are not available. However, studies have shown that the risk for childhood-onset malignancy is exceedingly high. In one study, 22 of 23 (96%) children with CMMRD had a diagnosis of cancer by the age of 18, and multiple individuals had three and even four metachronous tumors.[4]

The most commonly observed cancers are as follows:
- Gastrointestinal cancers. Colorectal and small bowel carcinomas can develop in childhood, adolescence, or early adulthood. It is not uncommon to have multiple synchronous or metachronous primary tumors. Adenomatous polyps of the colon and small bowel are often observed, with the number of polyps ranging from very few to dozens. Gastric polyps are possible as well. Importantly, the development and progression of adenomatous polyps and cancers seems to be very rapid in CMMRD.[5]
- Brain tumors. In one study of 22 individuals with CMMRD with a history of 40 tumors among them, 19 (48%) were brain tumors, making it the most common neoplasm. The spectrum of tumors reported included astrocytoma, glioblastoma multiforme, primitive neuroectodermal tumors, and medulloblastoma. Several low-grade gliomas were observed as well.[1]
- Hematologic malignancies. All major forms of leukemia and lymphomas have been reported in CMMRD, but lymphoid malignancies appear to be the most common.[1]
- Other traditional Lynch syndrome–related cancers have also been reported, including several uterine cancers in young adult women. Other rare, early-onset cancers have also been reported.[3]

Children with CMMRD often present with café au lait macules, and other features of neurofibromatosis type 1 (NF1), such as Lisch nodules, axillary freck-ling, and plexiform neurofibromas, have also been reported. The café au lait macules in CMMRD tend to be more diffuse and have irregular borders compared with those truly associated with NF1. It is important that clinicians are aware of the possibility for CMMRD when evaluating a child with skin manifestations sus-picious for NF1 as the consequences of misdiagnosis are dire.[1]

Interestingly, the family histories of children with CMMRD are not always as significant for Lynch syndrome–related cancers as one would expect, given that both par-ents are heterozygous for an MMR germline mutation. One theory is that heterozygous mutations in *MSH6* or *PMS2* are less common in Lynch syndrome and cause lower can-cer risks compared with mutations in *MLH1* and *MSH2*. However, CMMRD due to mutations in *MSH6* or *PMS2* does not appear to be less severe compared with CMMRD due to mutations in other MMR genes.[4]

Analysis of the MMR genes is clinically available in many laboratories and can detect homozygous or compound heterozygous mutations present in indi-viduals with CMMRD. It is also important to note that, although microsatellite analysis is a common screen-ing tool for microsatellite instability in colon and endometrial tumors when there is suspicion for Lynch syndrome, studies have shown that this analysis lacks sensitivity and specificity when evaluating for CMMRD. Immunohistochemistry analysis for the MMR proteins is the preferred screening tool, with one study showing 100% sensitivity and specificity on 26 CMMRD-related tumors.[4]

Suggested screening guidelines for individuals with CMMRD have been published by the International BMMRD Consortium and the European Consortium "Care for CMMR-D."[1,6]

## DICER1 SYNDROME

*DICER1* syndrome, also known as *DICER1*-pleuropul-monary blastoma familial tumor predisposition syn-drome or as pleuropulmonary blastoma (PPB) familial tumor and dysplasia syndrome, is a hereditary cancer syndrome that causes increased risk of several rare tumor types that can present at young ages. This is a relatively newly described syndrome. The link between familial PPB and *DICER1* mutations was discovered in 2009.[7] It is an autosomal dominant condition caused by mutations in the DICER1 gene, located at 14q32.13.[8] The hallmark tumor of this syndrome is PPB, which can present as early as infancy and usually before the age of 6 years.[9] Many other rare childhood and some

adult-onset tumors are observed as well. Importantly, it seems that the penetrance of *DICER1* mutations is low, meaning most individuals with a *DICER1* mutation never develop a *DICER1*-related tumor.[10] It should also be noted that the clinical presentation of adults with *DICER1* mutations is not yet well described.

The following are the tumors known to be part of the *DICER1* syndrome:

- PPB
- Ovarian sex cord-stromal tumors (Sertoli-Leydig cell tumor, juvenile granulosa cell tumor, and gynandro-blastoma)
- Cystic nephroma
- Thyroid gland neoplasia, including multinodular goiter (MNG), adenomas, or differentiated thyroid cancer
- Ciliary body medulloepithelioma
- Botryoid-type embryonal rhabdomyosarcoma of the cervix or other sites
- Nasal chondromesenchymal hamartoma
- Pituitary blastoma
- Pineoblastoma

Other tumors have also been reported, including Wilms tumor, neuroblastoma, and other childhood cancers.[9] As with all hereditary cancer syndromes, clini-cal presentation is variable both within and between families. Although, in many cases, PPB is the initial tumor that leads to a diagnosis, some families with *DICER1* syndrome have no reported cases of PPB.[10]

Analysis of the *DICER1* gene is clinically available, and it is expected that approximately 65% of individu-als with a personal history of PPB will have a muta-tion identified by sequencing of the gene.[11] At least one family with a large deletion in the *DICER1* gene and presentation consistent with the condition has been reported.[12] It is currently thought that approxi-mately 80% of *DICER1* mutations are inherited from an affected parent, whereas 20% are the result of a de novo event.[11]

As this is a newly described syndrome, there are no published surveillance guidelines available yet. How-ever, based on information from the International PPB Registry, the authors of the GeneReviews *DICER1*-Related Disorders entry have made recommendations for initial screenings and symptom-based imaging and laboratory studies for individuals with *DICER1* syndrome.[9]

## FAMILIAL ADENOMATOUS POLYPOSIS

Familial adenomatous polyposis (FAP) is a heredi-tary condition that results in significant adenomatous polyposis of the colon and increased risk of several cancers and benign tumors in childhood and throughout the lifetime. It is an autosomal dominant condition caused by mutations in the *APC* gene, located at 5q22.2.[13] The first sign of the condition is often early polyposis development in the colon, but benign or malignant extracolonic tumors in early childhood may develop prior to this.

According to the National Comprehensive Cancer Network (NCCN), testing for an *APC* mutation should be considered when an individual presents with 20 or more adenomatous colon polyps or when there is a known *APC* mutation in the family. Testing may also be considered for an individual presenting with a desmoid tumor, hepatoblastoma, cribriform-morular variant of papillary thyroid cancer, multifocal or bilateral congenital hypertrophy of the retinal pigment epithelium (CHRPE), or between 10 and 20 colon adenomas, depending on the age of onset, family history, and other clinical history of the individual.[14]

In classic FAP, the adenomatous polyps of the colon most often begin to develop in adolescence, with an average age of 16 years and a range of 7–36 years.[15] Without intervention (removal of the colon), colon cancer is inevitable with an average age of diagnosis of 39 years. Approximately 7% of individuals with classic FAP and their colons intact will develop a colon cancer by the age of 21 years.[16] Extracolonic cancer risks include the following:

- Small bowel carcinoma 4%–12%
- Thyroid cancer (mostly papillary) 1%–12%
- Hepatoblastoma, onset <5 years 1.6%
- Pancreatic cancer 1%
- Gastric cancer <1%
- Central nervous system (usually medulloblastoma) <1%
- Bile duct carcinoma, low, but elevated risk[17]

Other nonmalignant manifestations of FAP include osteomas, desmoid tumors, epidermoid cysts, fibromas, gastric and small bowel adenomas, supernumerary/missing teeth, and CHRPE.[14]

Analysis of the *APC* gene is clinically available. The detection rate with sequencing and deletion/duplication analysis is highest in individuals with a classic FAP phenotype who also have affected family members. Those with attenuated FAP phenotypes have much lower detection rates.[18] The rate of de novo mutations is estimated to be 20%–25%.[19] It should be noted that significant variation in the clinical presentation of FAP exists, even among family members carrying the same *APC* mutation. Although much information regarding genotype-phenotype correlations is now

known, management of individuals cannot be solely based on their genotype at this time.[20]

There are published clinical management guidelines for children and adults with FAP. See the NCCN FAP management guidelines.[14]

## FAMILIAL NEUROBLASTOMA

Familial neuroblastoma is an early childhood-onset condition that causes an increased risk of neuroblastic tumors, including neuroblastoma, ganglioneuroblastoma, and ganglioneuroma. This autosomal dominant condition can be caused by mutations in the *ALK* oncogene, located at 2p23.2-p23.1, or the *PHOX2B* gene at 4p13.[21] The main feature of germline *ALK* mutations is an increased risk of neuroblastic tumors. Those with *PHOX2B* mutations have an increased risk of neuroblastic tumors as well as disorders of neural crest development, which can include Hirschsprung disease, decreased esophageal motility, and congenital central hypoventilation syndrome.[22] Dysmorphic features, such as downslanting palpebral fissures, small nose, triangular shaped mouth, or low-set, posteriorly rotated ears, can also be observed.[23]

While consensus recommendations for when to test for *ALK* or *PHOX2B* mutations have yet to be published, some have recommended consideration of testing in the following situations:

- All children with somatic *ALK* pathogenic variants within a neuroblastic tumor
- An individual with a neuroblastic tumor who has at least one first-degree relative with a neuroblastic tumor
- An individual with a neuroblastic tumor and a personal/family history of a neural crest disorder, such as Hirschsprung disease or central hypoventilation syndrome, suggesting a *PHOX2B* mutation
- A simplex case (only affected individual in a family) with bilateral neuroblastoma or multifocal primary neuroblastic tumors[23]

Children with *ALK* mutations can develop any of the three types of neuroblastic tumors, and multiple primary tumors are possible. Neuroblastoma typically behaves as a more malignant tumor, whereas ganglioneuroma is more benign in nature. Ganglioneuroblastomas can display benign or malignant behavior.[23] The age of onset of these tumors is typically at younger ages than their sporadic counterparts (9 months vs. 2–3 years).[24]

Analysis of the *ALK* and *PHOX2B* genes is clinically available. Sequencing of the *ALK* gene is thought to detect a mutation in up to 80% of cases of familial neuroblastoma, whereas the detection of a germline mutation in simplex cases is rarer. *De novo* mutations in *ALK* have been reported, but the frequency of such events is unknown at this time. It is known that *ALK* mutations have reduced penetrance as several unaffected parents have been found to carry the same germline *ALK* mutation as their affected child.[25] Data are very limited, but one review of 10 families with *ALK* mutations reported that the overall penetrance of *ALK* mutations was 57%.[26]

As this is a very rare and relatively newly described condition, data are limited with regard to the best screening protocol for individuals with *ALK* and *PHOX2B* mutations. Published guidelines are not available yet. Some experts suggest physical examination, abdominal ultrasound, and urine catecholamine screening every 1–2 months in the first year of life and then every 3–4 months until age 10 years. Because of the risk for multiple primary tumors, children who have been successfully treated for neuroblastoma should continue the screening protocol.[23]

## HEREDITARY PARAGANGLIOMA-PHEOCHROMOCYTOMA SYNDROMES

Hereditary paraganglioma-pheochromocytoma (PGL/PCC) syndromes are conditions that cause an increased risk to develop PGLs and PCCs in childhood and throughout the lifetime. There are several subtypes of this condition (described below), characterized by the causative gene. PGLs are tumors that develop in the neuroendocrine tissues distributed along the paravertebral axis from the skull base to the pelvis. PCCs are PGLs that develop in the adrenal medulla. PGLs can be either sympathetic (they hypersecrete catecholamines) or parasympathetic (they are nonsecretory). PGLs of the head, neck, and upper mediastinum are typically parasympathetic, whereas PGLs of the lower mediastinum, abdomen, and pelvis (including PCCs) are typically sympathetic. PGLs and PCCs are typically diagnosed because of the mass effect of the tumor itself or symptoms from the hypersecretion of catecholamines (hypertension, headache, episodic profuse sweating, significant palpitations, pallor, and apprehension or anxiety).[27]

A hereditary PGL/PCC syndrome should be suspected in all individuals with a PGL or PCC, particularly in the following situations:

- Individuals with tumors that are:
  - Multiple, including bilateral PCC
  - Multifocal with multiple synchronous or metachronous tumors

- Recurrent
- Onset before age 45 years
- Individuals with a personal history of a PGL or PCC with a family history of either tumor type[28]

Subtypes of PGL/PCC include the following:

- PGL1 is caused by mutations in the *SDHD* gene at 11q23.1. These are autosomal dominant mutations with a paternal parent-of-origin effect, meaning those who inherit a mutation from their father have a high risk for development of PGL/PCC and those who inherit a mutation from their mother have a low, but not absent, risk for tumor development. Parasympathetic PGLs of the head and neck are the most common manifestation of PGL1, and the risk of malignancy is thought to be <5%.

- PGL2 is caused by mutations in the *SDHAF2* gene at 11q12.2. These are autosomal dominant mutations that also show evidence of a paternal parent-of-origin effect. Multiple PGLs of the head and neck are the most common presentation of *SDHAF2* mutation, and the risk of malignancy is low.

- PGL3 is caused by mutations in the *SDHC* gene at 1q23.3. These are rare autosomal dominant mutations. Parasympathetic PGLs of the head and neck are the most common manifestation of PGL3, and the risk of malignancy is thought to be low.

- PGL4 is caused by mutations in the *SDHB* gene at 1p36.13. These are autosomal dominant mutations. Individuals with *SDHB* mutations have higher risks for sympathetic extraadrenal PGLS and PCCs. Parasympathetic PGLs of the head and neck also occur. The risk for malignancy for those with *SDHB* mutations is high.

- PGL5 is caused by mutations in the *SDHA* gene at 5p15.33. These are autosomal dominant mutations and account for a small proportion of PGL/PCC. PGLs and PCCs can be observed, and the risk of malignancy is low.[27]

Other tumor types can also appear in individuals with *SDHx* mutations. Those with a PGL and GI stromal tumor are said to have Carney-Stratakis syndrome.[29] Thyroid and renal cell carcinomas have also been associated with *SDHB* and *SDHD* mutations.[30] Other genes are known to primarily cause increased risks for PCCs, including *MAX* and *TMEM127*.[31,32]

Of note, several different hereditary syndromes can also cause an increased risk of PGL or PCC, including neurofibromatosis type 1, multiple endocrine neoplasia type 1 (rare PCCs), multiple endocrine neoplasia type 2, von Hippel-Lindau syndrome, and Carney triad. These conditions need to be considered in the differential as well when a patient presents with PGL or PCC.[28]

Analysis of each of the genes associated with PGL/PCC is clinically available. Over the years there have been multiple genetic testing algorithms developed based on presentation of the individual (location of the PGL/PCC, biochemical results, etc.) and his/her family history. One such algorithm can be reviewed in Lenders et al.[28] However, with the availability of next-generation sequencing technology, many laboratories now offer PGL/PCC panels that include analysis of multiple genes associated with PGL/PCC, which can be more efficient and cost-effective than sequential gene-by-gene analysis.

Published clinical management guidelines for individuals with PGL/PCC are available from the Endocrine Society.[28] Although no consensus guidelines for the type, frequency, and age to begin screening for individuals with PGL/PCC have been published, suggested protocols can be reviewed in Timmers et al.[33] and the Hereditary Paraganglioma-Pheochromocytoma Syndromes entry on GeneReviews.[27]

## HERITABLE RETINOBLASTOMA

Heritable retinoblastoma (Rb) is a hereditary cancer syndrome that causes a significant increased risk of Rb as well as other tumors in childhood and adulthood. This is an autosomal dominant condition caused by mutations in the *RB1* gene, located at 13q14.2.[34] Rb is typically diagnosed prior to the age of 5 years. It presents as a unilateral tumor with no known family history in 60% of cases, with bilateral tumors and no known family history in 30% of cases, and with unilateral or bilateral tumors and a known family history in the remaining 10% of cases.[35]

A diagnosis of heritable Rb should be suspected in any individual who presents with Rb, retinoma (a benign retinal tumor), or with a family history of Rb.[35] The American Society of Clinical Oncologists has considered testing for a germline *RB1* mutation to be the standard of care for individuals with concerning personal and/or family histories for over 20 years.[36]

Cancer risks for individuals with an *RB1* mutation include the following:

- Retinoblastoma. The vast majority of families with *RB1* mutations show nearly complete penetrance, with relatives who have inherited the familial mutation almost always developing Rb. Fewer than 10% of families with heritable *RB1* have a low-penetrance mutation with a preponderance of unilateral Rb or no tumor development at all.[35]
- Pinealoblastomas. These rare and typically fatal tumors occur in the "retina-like" tissue of the pineal gland in the brain in approximately 5% of children with heritable Rb. Rare occurrences of primitive neuroectodermal tumor in nonpineal tissue have also been reported. If an individual develops either of these lesions, the term trilateral Rb is used.[37]
- Second primary tumors. There are also increased risks for specific types of secondary neoplasms in childhood/adolescence and in adulthood for individuals with heritable Rb. Osteosarcomas, soft tissue sarcomas, and melanomas are most common. Other studies have also found an increased incidence of lung, bladder, and other epithelial cancers. Although those who had external beam radiation therapy to treat a prior Rb do have higher risks for these secondary neoplasms, treatment-effect alone does not fully account for the increased risks.[35,38]

Analysis of the *RB1* gene is clinically available and it is currently estimated that up to 90% of individuals with heritable Rb will have a mutation detected. Individuals who present with bilateral Rb with or without a family history of the condition have a very high chance to have a mutation identified (virtually 100%). Individuals who present with unifocal Rb and no known family history of the disease have a much lower chance to carry a germline *RB1* mutation (approximately 14%). Additionally, 5%–7.5% of individuals who present with Rb with no known family history of the condition can have a deletion of chromosome region 13q14, which involves either a significant portion of or the entire *RB1* gene.[35] These individuals can often present with other developmental delays and birth defects.[39]

Guidelines for the management and surveillance of individuals with Rb and/or *RB1* mutations have been published by the Canadian Retinoblastoma Society. Suggestions are also made for the long-term follow-up of Rb survivors because those with *RB1* mutations are at significant increased risks for subsequent cancers.[40]

## JUVENILE POLYPOSIS SYNDROME

Juvenile polyposis syndrome (JPS) is a hereditary cancer syndrome that affects the GI system. Juvenile polyps, a type of hamartomatous polyp, can form in the stomach, small intestine, colon, and rectum.[41] Importantly, the term juvenile refers to the type of polyp, not the age of onset. Although polyps can develop in childhood and may be recognized because of resulting GI bleeding and/or anemia, cancers that develop because of JPS are typically of adult-onset (often with a younger age of onset than sporadic cancers).[42]

Clinical diagnostic criteria for JPS include the following:

- Individual with five or more juvenile polyps of the colorectum
- Individual with multiple juvenile polyps of the GI tract
- Individual with any number of juvenile polyps and a family history of juvenile polyps[41]

JPS is a condition with locus heterogeneity. It can be caused by mutations in the *BMPR1A* or *SMAD4* genes. It has been suggested that mutations in the *ENG* gene can also result in JPS, but there is not enough data at this time to confirm.[43] Importantly, most individuals with a *SMAD4* mutation will also develop features of hereditary hemorrhagic telangiectasia (HHT), resulting in a combined syndrome known as JPS/HHT.[44] It is vitally important that individuals with *SMAD4* mutations be screened for the manifestations of HHT beginning very early in life (see HHT guidelines below).

There can be great variability in the number of juvenile polyps that develop in JPS, even within the same family. While most individuals will develop some polyps by the age of 20, some will only have a few polyps and others may develop more than 100 over the lifetime.[42] Rarely, this condition presents as juvenile polyposis of infancy, and polyps develop in the first few months or years of life. This results in symptoms such as diarrhea, hemorrhage, failure to thrive, and intussusception.[41]

Although most juvenile polyps are benign, malignant transformation can occur. Estimated cancer risk for individuals with JPS include up to 50% risk for colon cancer and 21% risk for gastric cancer (if multiple polyps are present). Cancers of the pancreas and small intestine are rare in JPS but can occur at frequencies higher than the general population.[42]

Analysis of the *BMPR1A* and *SMAD4* genes is clinically available. Approximately 20%–25% of individuals with a JPS phenotype will have an identifiable mutation *BMPR1A* and 20% will have a mutation in *SMAD4*.[45] Again, those with *SMAD4* mutations are also at risk for HHT and will need to follow management guidelines for that condition as well beginning in early childhood. The rate of de novo cases of JPS is ~25%.[42]

There are published clinical management guidelines for children and adults with JPS and JPS/HHT. See the NCCN JPS management guidelines as well as HHT Foundation International's Guidelines Working Group publication.[14,46]

## LI-FRAUMENI SYNDROME

Li-Fraumeni syndrome (LFS) is a hereditary cancer syndrome with significant increased risk of malignancies in the pediatric population as well as into adulthood. It is an autosomal dominant condition caused by mutations in the *TP53* gene located at 17p13.[47] There are several cancer types that make up the core phenotype of the condition, including soft tissue sarcomas, osteosarcomas, early-onset breast cancers, brain tumors, adrenocortical carcinomas, and leukemias.[48] However, beyond this, many other malignancies are seen at higher frequencies than in the general population.[49]

There are multiple scenarios when analysis of the *TP53* gene is recommended:

- Classic LFS is defined as a proband with a sarcoma before age 45 who has a first-degree relative with any cancer before age 45 *and* another first- or second-degree relative with any cancer before age 45 or a sarcoma at any age.[50]
- The Chompret criteria include a proband with a cancer belonging to the LFS tumor spectrum (e.g., soft tissue sarcoma, osteosarcoma, brain tumor, premenopausal breast cancer, adrenocortical carcinoma, leukemia, lung bronchoalveolar cancer) before age 46 years *and* at least one first- or second-degree relative with an LFS tumor (except breast cancer if the proband has breast cancer) before age 56 years or with multiple tumors; *or*
- Proband with multiple tumors (except multiple breast tumors), two of which belong to the LFS tumor spectrum and the first of which occurred before age 46 years; *or*
- Proband with adrenocortical carcinoma or choroid plexus tumor, regardless of family history[51]
- Any woman diagnosed with breast cancer prior to age 30 who does not carry a pathogenic mutation in the *BRCA1* or *BRCA2* gene[52]

Estimated cancer risks for individuals with LFS are exceedingly high throughout the lifetime. Approximately 50% of individuals will develop a cancer by the age of 30 and 90% by the age of 60.[53] The most common type of sarcoma in those with LFS is a rhabdomyosarcoma with the onset prior to the age of 5 years.[54] The median age of brain tumors in LFS is 16 years. This can include astrocytoma, glioblastoma, medulloblastoma, and choroid plexus carcinoma.[55] Individuals with LFS are also at significant increased risk of multiple primary cancers over the lifetime. Estimates place the risk for a second and even third primary cancer at 57% and 38%, respectively, with survivors of childhood cancers having the highest risks for subsequent diagnoses.[56]

Analysis of the *TP53* gene is clinically available, and it is currently estimated that approximately 80% of individuals with LFS will have a mutation identified on sequencing or deletion/duplication analysis.[57] The rate of de novo mutations is estimated to be between 7% and 20%.[58]

There are published clinical management guidelines for children and adults with LFS syndrome, and it should be noted that these are evolving rapidly as more research is completed. See the NCCN LFS management guidelines as well as the surveillance strategy known as the Toronto Protocol.[48,59]

## MULTIPLE ENDOCRINE NEOPLASIA TYPE 1

Multiple endocrine neoplasia type 1 (MEN1) is a hereditary syndrome that causes significant increased risks for many different types of tumors throughout the lifetime. This is an autosomal dominant condition caused by mutations in the *MEN1* gene, located at 11q13.1.[60] Over 20 types of endocrine and nonendocrine tumors, some of which have malignant potential, have been described in MEN1, and reports of childhood-onset tumors have been well-documented.[61]

Clinical diagnostic criteria for MEN1 include the following:
- An individual with endocrine tumors from at least two of the three MEN1-related endocrine tumor categories (parathyroid, pituitary, or gastroenteropancreatic [GEP] tract)
- An individual with one MEN1-related endocrine tumor who has a first-degree relative with a clinical diagnosis of MEN1
- An individual with one MEN1-related endocrine tumor and a known *MEN1* gene mutation[62]

The main endocrine tumors seen in MEN1 include parathyroid tumors, pituitary tumors, GEP tract tumors, carcinoid tumors, and adrenocortical tumors.
- Parathyroid tumors manifesting as primary hyperparathyroidism are the first clinical sign of MEN1 in approximately 90% of cases. Most individuals will show signs of this by the age of 20–25 and virtually all are affected by age 50.[61] Although there have been several case reports of parathyroid carcinoma in individuals with MEN1, an increased risk of this malignancy is not thought to be a major feature of the condition.[63]
- Pituitary tumors are the first clinical sign of MEN1 in 10% of familial cases and 25% of simplex cases. They are found in 15%–50% of individuals with MEN1 and can occur as early as 5 years of age. Pituitary tumors that secrete prolactin (prolactinomas) are the most commonly observed subtype. Other tumors can secrete growth hormone alone, growth hormone and prolactin, thyroid-stimulating hormone, or adrenocorticotropic hormone. Clinical symptoms, including hyperprolactinemia, acromegaly, and Cushing syndrome, can result depending on the type of hormone that is secreted. Nonfunctioning pituitary adenomas occur as well.[62] Malignant transformation of pituitary tumors is not a common occurrence in MEN1.[64]
- Well-differentiated endocrine tumors of the GEP tract are present in 30%–70% of individuals with MEN1, with the most common secreting form being gastrinoma, which present in approximately 40% of cases.[62] These tumors are most commonly found in the duodenum, and the excess gastrin secretions manifest as Zollinger-Ellison syndrome. Gastrinomas are usually malignant, and half have already metastasized at the time of diagnosis.[61] Other secreting GEP endocrine tumors include insulinomas, glucagonomas, VIPomas. Insulinomas are typically benign, whereas glucagonomas and VIPomas are often malignant with frequent metastasis to the liver.[64] Nonfunctioning pancreatic neuroendocrine tumors (NETs) are very common in MEN1 as well with up to 55% of affected individuals having at least one tumor.[65] These can develop as early as adolescence and are increasingly recognized as the most common cause of death for individuals with MEN1.[62]
- Carcinoid tumors of the thymus, bronchus, and type II gastric enterochromaffin-like carcinoid tumors can be present in approximately 10% of individuals with MEN1. They are typically nonfunctioning tumors with later ages of onset. Thymic carcinoids are much more prevalent in males than females and can be particularly aggressive. Carcinoids of the bronchus are more prevalent in females and are less aggressive.[64]
- Adrenocortical tumors are observed in 20%–40% of individuals with MEN1 and are typically nonfunctioning. Less than 10% secrete hormones, which may include aldosterone and cortisol. PCCs are rare in MEN1 (<1%).[62] Malignant transformation of adrenocortical tumors is also rare, but the risk does increase with the size of the tumor.[66]

The nonendocrine tumors/lesions that can present in MEN1 include lipomas (30%), facial angiofibromas (up to 85%), collagenomas (up to 70%), ependymomas (rare), meningiomas (8%), and leiomyomas.[62,64]

Analysis of the *MEN1* gene is clinically available, and it is currently estimated that over 90% of familial cases of MEN1 will have a detectable mutation on sequencing and deletion/duplication analysis of the *MEN1* gene.[67] The mutation detection rate in simplex cases of MEN1 is significantly lower at approximately 65%.[68] The rate of de novo germline *MEN1* mutations is estimated to be 10%.[69]

There are published clinical management and surveillance guidelines for children and adults with MEN1. Biochemical screening and imaging for some tumors begins as early as 5 years of age. See the Clinical Practice Guideline for Multiple Endocrine Neoplasia Type 1.[62]

## MULTIPLE ENDOCRINE NEOPLASIA TYPE 2

Multiple endocrine neoplasia type 2 (MEN2) is a hereditary cancer syndrome that causes significant increased risk of medullary thyroid carcinoma (MTC) beginning at young ages. It is an autosomal dominant condition caused by mutations in the *RET* protooncogene, located at 10q11.21.[70] There are three main subtypes of MEN2: MEN2A, familial medullary thyroid carcinoma (FMTC), and MEN2B.

- MEN2A accounts for approximately 70%–80% of cases of MEN2. Individuals with this subtype have a 95% risk for MTC, a 50% risk for PCC, and a 20%–30% risk for hyperparathyroidism (adenoma/hyperplasia).[71] A clinical diagnosis of MEN2A is given when two or more tumor types are present in one individual or close relatives.
- FMTC accounts for approximately 10%–20% of cases of MEN2. The clinical definition of FMTC is at least four family members with MTC in the absence of PCC or parathyroid disease. However, caution must be taken to not prematurely give a diagnosis of FMTC to a kindred if the presence of a PCC or parathyroid disease for any individual has not been carefully excluded. Some experts think of FMTC as a variant of MEN2A with the later onset of MTC and lower penetrance for other MEN2A tumors.[72]
- MEN2B accounts for approximately 5% of cases of MEN2. Individuals with this subtype have a virtually 100% risk for an aggressive form of MTC at a very young age. There is also a 50% risk for development of PCC, and parathyroid disease is absent. Infants and children with MEN2B often presents with other clinical findings, including marfanoid habitus, ganglioneuromatosis of the GI tract and oral mucosa, and medullated corneal nerve fibers.[73]

Of note, germline mutations in the *RET* gene can also cause Hirschsprung disease and are found in approximately 50% of familial cases and 35% of simplex cases.[74] Those with *RET* mutations affecting exon 10 can often have cosegregation of Hirschsprung disease and MEN2A/FMTC in the same individual or family.[72]

Analysis of the *RET* gene is clinically available, and it is estimated that detection rates are >98%, >95%, and >98% for MEN2A, FMTC, and MEN2B, respectively.[72,75] The rate of de novo mutations in MEN2A is thought to be ≤5%, whereas the rate for MEN2B cases is 50%.[72] Genetic testing is recommended for all individuals who present with MTC (or primary C-cell hyperplasia), even if there is no known family history of the condition. Approximately 25%–30% of individuals with MTC will carry a *RET* mutation. One study showed that ~7% of individuals with apparently simplex cases of MTC carried a germline mutation.[76]

A great deal has been learned about the appropriate medical management for individuals with MEN2 using genotype-phenotype correlations. Although preventive total thyroidectomy is necessary for all (sometimes within the first year of life), the timing of this can often be directed by the particular codon of the *RET* gene that is affected. Biochemical screening for other features of MEN2 can also be directed by the codon involved. See the Medullary Thyroid Cancer: Management Guidelines of the American Thyroid Association report for further details.[72]

## NEUROFIBROMATOSIS TYPE 2

Neurofibromatosis type 2 (NF2) is a hereditary condition that causes a predisposition to the development of schwannomas of the bilateral vestibular nerves. Schwannomas can also develop in other cranial, spinal, and peripheral nerves. Other tumors types, such as ependymomas, astrocytomas, and meningiomas, as well as ocular and skin manifestations, can also be observed.[77] It is an autosomal dominant syndrome caused by mutations in the *NF2* gene, located at 22q12.2.[78]

Features of NF2 can include the following:

- Vestibular schwannoma for the vast majority, with symptoms of tinnitus, balance dysfunction, and/or hearing loss[77]
- Spinal tumors, including schwannomas, meningiomas, and astrocytomas[79]
- Meningiomas can be intracranial or spinal[80]
- Ocular findings, including posterior subcapsular lens opacities, cataract, and retinal or pigment hamartomas[79]
- Skin findings can include NF2 plaques, cutaneous and nodular schwannomas, and a small number of café au lait macules[79]
- Mononeuropathy in childhood (facial palsy, squint, or hand/foot drop) and polyneuropathy in adulthood[81,82]

Traditionally, NF2 was considered an adult-onset disease, but it is increasingly recognized that clinical features do present in childhood, and the course of the condition can vary greatly from the adult-onset form. A congenital form of the condition with onset of bilateral vestibular schwannoma in infancy has been described. The clinical presentation also appears to differ between individuals with onset of symptoms prior to puberty and those with symptoms beginning in adolescence. See Ruggieri et al.[79] for a detailed review of pediatric presentations of NF2.

There have been several iterations of diagnostic criteria for NF2 throughout the years. The most recent updates have made adjustments to allow for diagnosis at younger ages, especially for those with founder mutations.[79] The Baser criteria for diagnosis of NF2 were most recently updated in 2011. These criteria use a point system, which takes into account family history, clinical symptoms of NF2, and the age of onset. It helps guide clinicians as to when to consider *NF2* molecular testing and differentiating between possible NF2, mosaic NF2, and confirmed constitutional NF2.[83]

Analysis of the *NF2* gene is clinically available, and the detection rate can exceed 90% for familial cases when sequencing and deletion/duplication methods are used.[84] It is thought that approximately 50% of cases of NF2 arise because of a de novo mutation and that 25%–30% of these individuals have the condition as a result of somatic mosaicism.[85] Because of this, the detection rate for a mutation in simplex cases is lower than for familial cases. Analysis of tumor tissue may be helpful in identifying the causative mutation in individuals with suspected mosaicism.[86]

There are surveillance guidelines for individuals with NF2, which begin in childhood and focus on imaging to monitor for the development of intracranial tumors as well as hearing and eye examinations. Management of NF2 includes monitoring of asymptomatic tumors and surgical removal of others. There has also been a significant amount of research in recent years into pharmacologic therapies to help ease the tumor burden for individuals with NF2.[79]

## PEUTZ-JEGHERS SYNDROME

Peutz-Jeghers syndrome (PJS) is a hereditary cancer syndrome that is characterized by early-onset GI polyposis, abnormal mucocutaneous pigmentation, and increased cancer risks. This is an autosomal disorder caused by mutations in the *STK11* gene at 19p13.3.[87] The characteristic lesion of PJS is a specific PJS-type hamartomatous polyp, which is most frequently observed in the small intestine but can be observed throughout the GI tract and at extraintestinal sites as well.[88]

A clinical diagnosis of PJS can be made for an individual with one of the following:

- Two or more histologically confirmed PJS-type hamartomatous polyps
- Any number of PJS-type polyps detected in an individual with an affected close relative
- Characteristic mucocutaneous pigmentation in an individual with an affected close relative
- Any number of PJS-type polyps in an individual with characteristic mucocutaneous pigmentation[89]

The PJS-type hamartomatous polyps can cause significant nonmalignant issues, such as bleeding/anemia, bowel obstruction, and intussusception beginning in childhood. One study showed that by the age of 18, 68% of children with PJS had at least one emergency laparotomy.[90] It is important to note that other polyp types, particularly adenomas, can also be observed throughout the GI tract. Significant variability in the age of onset, number, and location of polyps can be observed both within and between families with PJS.[88]

The mucocutaneous hyperpigmentation observed in PJS includes dark blue/brown macules present around the mouth, nostrils, eyes, fingers, as well as the buccal mucosa and perianal area. These lesions are often present in infancy/early childhood and can fade after puberty and into adulthood, although the buccal mucosal lesions tend to remain.[91]

Rare gonadal tumors can be observed in females and males with PJS. Females are at risk for sex cord tumors with annular tubules (SCTATs) and mucinous tumors of the ovaries and fallopian tubes. The SCTATs in PJS are small, bilateral tumors with a usually benign course. Males can develop large-cell calcifying Sertoli cell tumors (LCSTs) of the testes at young ages.[92]

The risks of malignancy in PJS are significant and, on average, tumors are diagnosed at much younger ages than their sporadic counterparts. The following cancer risks were compiled by Syngal et al. (2015):

- Colon—39%, average age of diagnosis 42–46 years
- Gastric—29%, average age of diagnosis 30–40 years
- Small bowel—13%, average age of diagnosis 37–42 years
- Pancreatic—11%–36%, average age of diagnosis 41–52 years
- Breast (female)—32%–54%, average age of diagnosis 37–59 years
- Ovarian (mostly SCTATs)—21%, average age of diagnosis 28 years
- Cervix (adenoma malignum)—10%, average age of diagnosis 34–40 years
- Uterine—9%, average age of diagnosis 43 years

- Testicular (LCSTs)—9%, average age of diagnosis 6–9 years
- Lung—7%–17%, average age of diagnosis 47 years[93]

Analysis of the *STK11* gene is clinically available, and it is currently estimated that up to 96% of individuals with a clinical diagnosis of PJS will have a detectable mutation when sequencing and deletion/duplication methods are utilized.[94] Although there do seem to be a fair number of sporadic cases of PJS, the true de novo rate of *STK11* mutations is unknown at this time because of the potential that subtle clinical findings may go unnoticed in family members.[88]

There are published clinical management guidelines for children and adults with PJS, which focus on organ-specific polyp and tumor surveillance. See the NCCN PJS management guidelines for details.[14]

## PTEN HAMARTOMA TUMOR SYNDROME

*PTEN* hamartoma tumor syndrome (PHTS) is a hereditary condition that can cause significant increased risks for benign and malignant overgrowths. This is an autosomal dominant condition caused by mutations in the *PTEN* gene, located at 10q23.31.[95] PHTS includes four different clinical phenotypes: Cowden syndrome (CS), Bannayan-Riley-Ruvalcaba syndrome (BRRS), *PTEN*-related Proteus syndrome (PS), and Proteus-like syndrome.

CS is a complex condition with many clinical symptoms affecting various different organ systems. The possible features of CS are categorized into major and minor criteria and are regularly reviewed and updated by the NCCN. Over the years many iterations of genetic testing criteria and clinical diagnostic criteria have been established for CS.[59,96] An online scoring tool has also been developed to help clinicians estimate the chance that a patient carries a *PTEN* mutation.[97]

- Major criteria for CS include breast cancer, thyroid cancer (follicular), endometrial cancer (epithelial), ≥3 GI hamartomas, macrocephaly (>97%ile), Lhermitte-Duclos disease (adult), macular pigmentation of the glans penis, and multiple mucocutaneous lesions (≥3 trichilemmomas, ≥3 palmoplantar keratotic pits and/or acral hyperkeratotic papules, ≥3 mucocutaneous neuromas, *or* ≥3 oral papillomas).[59]
- Minor criteria for CS include autism spectrum disorder, colon cancer, esophageal glycogenic acanthoses, ≥3 lipomas, intellectual disability (IQ≤75), renal cell carcinoma, testicular lipomatosis, thyroid cancer (papillary or follicular variant of papillary),

thyroid structural lesions (adenoma, MNG), and vascular anomalies (including multiple intracranial developmental venous anomalies).[59]
- Cancer risks in CS include:
  - Female breast cancer—85% (50% penetrance by age 50)
  - Male breast cancer—increased according to some, but not all studies
  - Thyroid cancer—35% (the median age of diagnosis is 37, but childhood-onset reported)
  - Endometrial cancer—28% (risk beginning in the 30s and 40s)
  - Colon cancer—9% (risk begins in the late 30s, 90% have polyps of various types)
  - Renal cell carcinoma—35% (risk begins in 40s)
  - Melanoma—>5% (childhood-onset reported)[98]

BRRS is characterized by the main features of macrocephaly, hamartomatous intestinal polyposis, lipomas, and pigmented macules of the glans penis.[99] Other features can include high birth weight, developmental delays, intellectual disabilities, myopathy of the proximal muscles, joint hyperextensibility, pectus excavatum, and scoliosis.[100]

PS is a variable condition that seems to most often present in a mosaic pattern. *PTEN*-related PS is characterized by segmental overgrowth of tissues commonly affecting the skeleton, skin, adipose tissue, and central nervous system. This is progressive overgrowth, which begins to develop rapidly in early childhood and continues throughout life, causing disfigurement and other complications including increased risks for blood clots and pulmonary embolism. Proteus-like syndrome is not defined, but it is a name given to those individuals with findings consistent PS who do not meet the clinical criteria.[101]

Analysis of the *PTEN* gene is clinically available, and it is anticipated that up to 90% of individuals with CS will have an identifiable mutation when sequencing (including the promoter region) and deletion/duplication techniques are used. The detection rate for individuals with BRRS is expected to approach 70%. Those with Proteus-like syndrome and PS have mutations detected by sequencing analysis 50% and 20% of the time, respectively. The rate of de novo *PTEN* mutations in CS and BRRS is unknown, but simplex and familial cases have been reported. Almost all individuals with PS and Proteus-like syndrome are simplex cases.[101] For those with a clinical diagnosis of CS and no identifiable *PTEN* mutation the possibility of a germline *KLLN* epimutation, *SDHB*, *SDHC*, *SDHD*, *PIK3CA*, *AKT1*, or *SEC23B* could be considered.[102–105] However, this is controversial.

There are published clinical management guidelines for children and adults with CS/PHTS, and it should be noted that these are updated regularly as more research is completed. See the NCCN PHTS management guidelines.[59] Individuals with BRRS *and* a mutation in the *PTEN* gene are thought to have the same cancer risks as individuals with a diagnosis of CS (discussed above) and should follow the same screening guidelines. It is also suggested by experts in PHTS that clinicians consider following the CS cancer screening guidelines for their patients with PS and Proteus-like syndrome *and* a *PTEN* mutation.[101]

## RHABDOID TUMOR PREDISPOSITION SYNDROME 1

Rhabdoid tumor predisposition syndrome 1 (RTPS1) is a hereditary cancer syndrome associated with increased risk of rhabdoid tumors in infancy and early childhood. These are aggressive tumors that are referred to as atypical teratoid/rhabdoid tumors (AT/RTs) when present in the central nervous syndrome and referred to as malignant rhabdoid tumors (MRTs) when present in the kidney or other extrarenal sites.[106] RTPS1 is an autosomal dominant condition caused by mutations in the *SMARCB1* gene, located at 22q11.23.[107] Mutations in this gene can also cause hereditary schwannomatosis, and at least one family with presentation of both conditions has been reported.[108]

Of note, germline mutations in another gene have been implicated in association with predisposition to rhabdoid tumors. Rhabdoid tumor predisposition syndrome 2 (RTPS2) is caused by mutations in the *SMARCA4* gene located at 19p13.2 and results in an increased risk of AT/RTs and MRTs.[109]

The onset of rhabdoid tumors in RTPS1 is typically at very young ages, with the median age of diagnosis at 5 months in one study. This was younger than the median age of 18 months for those with sporadic rhabdoid tumors. Affected individuals can also develop multiple primary tumors, and treatment outcomes remain poor.[106]

Analysis of the *SMARCB1* gene is clinically available, and a recent study suggested that as many as 35% of rhabdoid tumors may be associated with germline mutations. Comprehensive analysis of the gene using direct sequencing, MLPA, and SNP array analysis is necessary to achieve the highest detection rates. Because of the rarity of the syndrome, data is quite limited, but inherited *SMARCB1* mutations, de novo mutations, and cases of germline mosaicism have been reported.[106]

Formal published surveillance guidelines for individuals with RTPS1 are not yet available. Clinicians with experience in managing RTPS1 have suggested brain MRIs and renal ultrasounds to monitor for tumor development in infancy and early childhood.[106,108] The potential for schwannoma development should also be discussed with individuals known to carry *SMARCB1* mutations.

## VON HIPPEL-LINDAU SYNDROME

Von Hippel-Lindau syndrome (VHL) is a complex hereditary condition that causes an increased risk of cysts, tumors, and malignancies of multiple different organ systems. This is an autosomal dominant condition caused by mutations in the *VHL* gene at location 3p25.3.[110] The hallmark findings of VHL are hemangioblastomas of the retina, brain, and spinal cord. Clear cell renal cell carcinoma, pancreatic NETs, PCC, multiple renal and pancreatic cysts, endolymphatic sac tumors, and epididymal and broad ligament cysts can be seen as well.[111]

A clinical diagnosis of VHL can be established in the three following situations:

1. A simplex case with *two or more* characteristic VHL lesions:
   - Two or more hemangioblastomas of the retina, spine, or brain or a single hemangioblastoma in association with a visceral manifestation (e.g., multiple kidney or pancreatic cysts)
   - Renal cell carcinoma
   - Adrenal or extraadrenal PCCs
   - Less commonly, endolymphatic sac tumors, papillary cystadenomas of the epididymis or broad ligament, or NETs of the pancreas
2. An individual with a family history of VHL and with *one or more* VHL lesions:
   - Retinal hemangioblastoma
   - Spinal or cerebellar hemangioblastoma
   - Adrenal or extraadrenal PCC
   - Renal cell carcinoma
   - Multiple renal and pancreatic cysts
   - Less commonly, endolymphatic sac tumors, papillary cystadenomas of the epididymis or broad ligament, or NETs of the pancreas
3. Identification of a germline *VHL* mutation confirms the diagnosis of VHL for a simplex or familial case regardless of the current clinical presentation.[112]

CNS hemangioblastomas are the cardinal feature of VHL and occur in 60%–80% of affected patients. They are the presenting symptom 40% of the time.[113] Retinal hemangioblastomas (sometimes called retinal angiomas) are the most common presenting symptom and often develop in childhood. Eventually, they are detected in almost 70% of individuals.[114] The lifetime risk for clear cell renal cell carcinoma approaches 70% and is a major cause of mortality in VHL. The average age of onset is ~40 years, and multiple primary tumors can develop. Renal cysts, which do not typically affect renal function, are also quite common.[113] PCCs (unilateral or bilateral) develop at an average of 30 years of age in approximately 10%–20% of patients.[114] Multiple pancreatic cysts are very common in VHL and rarely have an effect on pancreatic function. The more concerning pancreatic lesions are the NETs, which develop in 5%–17% of individuals.[111,113] Endolymphatic sac tumors present in 10%–16% of individuals, and the associated hearing loss and disequilibrium can sometimes be the initial presenting symptoms of VHL.[115] Epididymal or papillary cystadenomas are common in males with VHL and rarely have a clinical effect (bilateral lesions can cause infertility).[112]

Analysis of the *VHL* gene is clinically available, and it is expected that virtually 100% of individuals with the condition will have a detectable mutation when sequencing and deletion/duplication methods are used.[116] Newer studies quote a detection rate of >95%.[113] The rate of de novo mutations is estimated to be 20%, and the penetrance of the condition approaches 100% by the age of 65.[112,117] The American Society of Clinical Oncologists has suggested that testing for a germline *VHL* mutation be the standard of care for individuals with concerning personal and/or family histories for over 20 years.[36]

Early detection of potential manifestations of VHL is key to reducing disease-related morbidity and mortality.[113] Suggested surveillance guidelines have been developed by the VHL Alliance and are largely accepted throughout the world.[118]

## REFERENCES

1. Durno C, Sherman P, Aronson M, et al. Phenotypic and genotypic characterisation of biallelic mismatch repair deficiency (BMMR-D) syndrome. *Eur J Cancer.* 2015;51(8): 977–983. http://dx.doi.org/10.1016/j.ejca.2015.02.008.
2. Durno C, Aronson M, Tabori U, Malkin D, Gallinger S, Chan H. Oncologic surveillance for subjects with biallelic mismatch repair gene mutations: 10 year follow-up of a kindred. *Pediatr Blood Cancer.* 2011;59(4):652–656. http://dx.doi.org/10.1002/pbc.24019.
3. Wimmer K, Kratz C, Vasen H, et al. Diagnostic criteria for constitutional mismatch repair deficiency syndrome: suggestions of the European consortium 'Care for CM-MRD' (C4CMMRD). *J Med Genet.* 2014;51(6):355–365. http://dx.doi.org/10.1136/jmedgenet-2014-102284.
4. Bakry D, Aronson M, Durno C, et al. Genetic and clinical determinants of constitutional mismatch repair deficiency syndrome: report from the constitutional mismatch repair deficiency consortium. *Eur J Cancer.* 2014;50(5):987–996. http://dx.doi.org/10.1016/j.ejca.2013.12.005.
5. Aronson M, Gallinger S, Cohen Z, et al. Gastrointestinal findings in the largest series of patients with hereditary biallelic mismatch repair deficiency syndrome: report from the International Consortium. *Am J Gastroenterol.* 2016;111(2):275–284. http://dx.doi.org/10.1038/ajg.2015.392.
6. Vasen H, Ghorbanoghli Z, Bourdeaut F, et al. Guidelines for surveillance of individuals with constitutional mismatch repair-deficiency proposed by the European Consortium "Care for CMMR-D" (C4CMMR-D). *J Med Genet.* 2014;51(5):283–293. http://dx.doi.org/10.1136/jmedgenet-2013-102238.
7. Hill D, Ivanovich J, Priest J, et al. DICER1 mutations in familial pleuropulmonary blastoma. *Science.* 2009;325(5943):965. http://dx.doi.org/10.1126/science.1174334.
8. *OMIM Entry – # 601200-Pleuropulmonary Blastoma; PPB.* Omimorg; 2016. Available at: https://www.omim.org/entry/601200?search=dicer1&highlight=dicer1.
9. Doros L, Schultz KA, Stewart DR, et al. DICER1-related disorders. In: Pagon RA, Adam MP, Ardinger HH, et al., eds. *GeneReviews® [Internet].* Seattle, WA: University of Washington; April 24, 2014. 1993-2016. Available from: https://www.ncbi.nlm.nih.gov/books/NBK196157/.
10. Slade I, Bacchelli C, Davies H, et al. DICER1 syndrome: clarifying the diagnosis, clinical features and management implications of a pleiotropic tumour predisposition syndrome. *J Med Genet.* 2011;48(4):273–278. http://dx.doi.org/10.1136/jmg.2010.083790.
11. Hill DA, Wang JD, Schoettler P, et al. Germline DICER1 mutations are common in both hereditary and presumed sporadic pleuropulmonary blastoma [Abstract]. *Lab Invest.* 2010;90:311.
12. Sabbaghian N, Srivastava A, Hamel N, et al. Germ-line deletion in DICER1 revealed by a novel MLPA assay using synthetic oligonucleotides. *Eur J Hum Genet.* 2013;22(4):564–567. http://dx.doi.org/10.1038/ejhg.2013.215.
13. *OMIM Entry – # 175100-Familial Adenomatous Polyposis 1; FAP1.* Omimorg; 2016. Available at: https://www.omim.org/entry/175100?search=apc&highlight=apc.
14. National Comprehensive Cancer Network. Genetic/familial high-risk assessment: colorectal. *NCCN Clinical Practice Guidelines in Oncology. Version 2*; 2016. www.nccn.org.
15. Petersen GM, Slack J, Nakamura Y. Screening guidelines and premorbid diagnosis of familial adenomatous polyposis using linkage. *Gastroenterology.* 1991;100(6):1658–1664.
16. Bussey HJR. *Familial Polyposis Coli.* Johns Hopkins University Press; 1975.

17. Jasperson KW, Burt RW. APC-associated polyposis conditions. In: Pagon RA, Adam MP, Ardinger HH, et al., eds. *GeneReviews® [Internet]*. Seattle, WA: University of Washington; December 18, 1998. 1993-2016. Available from: https://www.ncbi.nlm.nih.gov/books/NBK1345/.

18. Sieber O, Lamlum H, Crabtree M, et al. Whole-gene APC deletions cause classical familial adenomatous polyposis, but not attenuated polyposis or "multiple" colorectal adenomas. *Proc Natl Acad Sci USA*. 2002;99(5):2954–2958. http://dx.doi.org/10.1073/pnas.042699199.

19. Bisgaard M, Fenger K, Bülow S, Niebuhr E, Mohr J. Familial adenomatous polyposis (FAP): frequency, penetrance, and mutation rate. *Hum Mutat*. 1994;3(2):121–125. http://dx.doi.org/10.1002/humu.1380030206.

20. Friedl W. Can APC mutation analysis contribute to therapeutic decisions in familial adenomatous polyposis? Experience from 680 FAP families. *Gut*. 2001;48(4):515–521. http://dx.doi.org/10.1136/gut.48.4.515.

21. *OMIM Entry – # 256700-Neuroblastoma, Susceptibility to.* Omimorg; 2016. Available at: https://www.omim.org/entry/256700.

22. Raabe E, Laudenslager M, Winter C, et al. Prevalence and functional consequence of PHOX2B mutations in neuroblastoma. *Oncogene*. 2007;27(4):469–476. http://dx.doi.org/10.1038/sj.onc.1210659.

23. Greengard EG, Park JR. ALK-related neuroblastic tumor susceptibility. In: Pagon RA, Adam MP, Ardinger HH, et al., eds. *GeneReviews® [Internet]*. Seattle, WA: University of Washington; January 5, 2010. 1993-2016. Available from: https://www.ncbi.nlm.nih.gov/books/NBK24599/.

24. Park J, Eggert A, Caron H. Neuroblastoma: biology, prognosis, and treatment. *Pediatr Clin N Am*. 2008;55(1):97–120. http://dx.doi.org/10.1016/j.pcl.2007.10.014.

25. Mossé Y, Laudenslager M, Longo L, et al. Identification of ALK as a major familial neuroblastoma predisposition gene. *Nature*. 2008;455(7215):930–935. http://dx.doi.org/10.1038/nature07261.

26. Eng C. Cancer: a ringleader identified. *Nature*. 2008;455(7215):883–884. http://dx.doi.org/10.1038/455883a.

27. Kirmani S, Young WF. Hereditary paraganglioma-pheochromocytoma syndromes. In: Pagon RA, Adam MP, Ardinger HH, et al., eds. *GeneReviews® [Internet]*. Seattle, WA: University of Washington; May 21, 2008. 1993-2016. Available from: https://www.ncbi.nlm.nih.gov/books/NBK1548/.

28. Lenders J, Duh Q, Eisenhofer G, et al. Pheochromocytoma and paraganglioma: an endocrine society clinical practice guideline. *J Clin Endocrinol Metab*. 2014;99(6):1915–1942. http://dx.doi.org/10.1210/jc.2014-1498.

29. Pasini B, McWhinney S, Bei T, et al. Clinical and molecular genetics of patients with the Carney–Stratakis syndrome and germline mutations of the genes coding for the succinate dehydrogenase subunits SDHB, SDHC, and SDHD. *Eur J Hum Genet*. 2007;16(1):79–88. http://dx.doi.org/10.1038/sj.ejhg.5201904.

30. Ricketts C, Forman J, Rattenberry E, et al. Tumor risks and genotype-phenotype-proteotype analysis in 358 patients with germline mutations in SDHB and SDHD. *Hum Mutat*. 2010;31(1):41–51. http://dx.doi.org/10.1002/humu.21136.

31. Burnichon N, Cascon A, Schiavi F, et al. MAX mutations cause hereditary and sporadic pheochromocytoma and paraganglioma. *Clin Cancer Res*. 2012;18(10):2828–2837. http://dx.doi.org/10.1158/1078-0432.ccr-12-0160.

32. Yao L, Schiavi F, Cascon A, et al. Spectrum and prevalence of FP/TMEM127 gene mutations in pheochromocytomas and paragangliomas. *JAMA*. 2010;304(23):2611. http://dx.doi.org/10.1001/jama.2010.1830.

33. Timmers H, Gimenez-Roqueplo A, Mannelli M, Pacak K. Clinical aspects of SDHx-related pheochromocytoma and paraganglioma. *Endocr Relat Cancer*. 2009;16(2):391–400. http://dx.doi.org/10.1677/erc-08-0284.

34. *OMIM Entry – # 180200-Retinoblastoma; RB1.* Omimorg; 2016. Available at: https://www.omim.org/entry/180200.

35. Lohmann DR, Gallie BL. Retinoblastoma. In: Pagon RA, Adam MP, Ardinger HH, et al., eds. *GeneReviews® [Internet]*. Seattle, WA: University of Washington; July 18, 2000. 1993-2016. Available from: https://www.ncbi.nlm.nih.gov/books/NBK1452/.

36. Statement of the American Society of Clinical Oncology. Genetic testing for cancer susceptibility. *J Clin Oncol*. 1996;14:1730–1736.

37. de Jong M, Kors W, de Graaf P, Castelijns J, Kivelä T, Moll A. Trilateral retinoblastoma: a systematic review and meta-analysis. *Lancet Oncol*. 2014;15(10):1157–1167. http://dx.doi.org/10.1016/s1470-2045(14)70336-5.

38. Marees T, van Leeuwen F, de Boer M, Imhof S, Ringens P, Moll A. Cancer mortality in long-term survivors of retinoblastoma. *Eur J Cancer*. 2009;45(18):3245–3253. http://dx.doi.org/10.1016/j.ejca.2009.05.011.

39. Mitter D, Ullmann R, Muradyan A, et al. Genotype–phenotype correlations in patients with retinoblastoma and interstitial 13q deletions. *Eur J Hum Genet*. 2011;19(9):947–958. http://dx.doi.org/10.1038/ejhg.2011.58.

40. Gallie B. Canadian guidelines for retinoblastoma care. *Can J Ophthalmol*. 2009;44(6):639–642. http://dx.doi.org/10.3129/i09-229.

41. Brosens L. Juvenile polyposis syndrome. *World J Gastroenterol*. 2011;17(44):4839. http://dx.doi.org/10.3748/wjg.v17.i44.4839.

42. Larsen Haidle J, Howe JR. Juvenile polyposis syndrome. In: Pagon RA, Adam MP, Ardinger HH, et al., eds. *GeneReviews® [Internet]*. Seattle, WA: University of Washington; May 13, 2003. 1993-2016. Available from: https://www.ncbi.nlm.nih.gov/books/NBK1469/.

43. Howe J, Haidle J, Lal G, et al. ENG mutations in MADH4/BMPR1A mutation negative patients with juvenile polyposis. *Clin Genet*. 2006;71(1):91–92. http://dx.doi.org/10.1111/j.1399-0004.2007.00734.x.

44. O'Malley M, LaGuardia L, Kalady M, et al. The prevalence of hereditary hemorrhagic telangiectasia in juvenile polyposis syndrome. *Dis Colon Rectum.* 2012;55(8):886–892. http://dx.doi.org/10.1097/dcr.0b013e31825aad32.

45. Sayed MG, Ahmed AF, Ringold JR, et al. Germline SMAD4 or BMPR1A mutations and phenotype of juvenile polyposis. *Ann Surg Oncol.* 2002;9(9):901–906.

46. Faughnan M, Palda V, Garcia-Tsao G, et al. International guidelines for the diagnosis and management of hereditary haemorrhagic telangiectasia. *J Med Genet.* 2009;48(2):73–87. http://dx.doi.org/10.1136/jmg.2009.069013.

47. *OMIM Entry – # 151623-Li-Fraumeni Syndrome 1; LFS1.* Omimorg; 2016. Available at: https://www.omim.org/entry/151623.

48. Villani A, Tabori U, Schiffman J, et al. Biochemical and imaging surveillance in germline TP53 mutation carriers with Li-Fraumeni syndrome: a prospective observational study. *Lancet Oncol.* 2011;12(6):559–567. http://dx.doi.org/10.1016/s1470-2045(11)70119-x.

49. Nichols KE, Malkin D, Garber JE, Fraumeni Jr JF, Li FP. Germ-line p53 mutations predispose to a wide spectrum of early-onset cancers. *Cancer Epidemiol Biomarkers Prev.* 2001;10(2):83–87.

50. Li FP, Fraumeni Jr JF, Mulvihill JJ, et al. A cancer family syndrome in twenty-four kindreds. *Cancer Res.* 1988;48(18):5358–5362.

51. Tinat J, Bougeard G, Baert-Desurmont S, et al. 2009 version of the Chompret criteria for Li Fraumeni syndrome. *J Clin Oncol.* 2009;27(26):e108–e109. http://dx.doi.org/10.1200/jco.2009.22.7967.

52. Schneider K, Zelley K, Nichols KE, et al. Li-Fraumeni syndrome. In: Pagon RA, Adam MP, Ardinger HH, et al., eds. *GeneReviews® [Internet].* Seattle, WA: University of Washington; January 19, 1999. 1993-2016. Available from: https://www.ncbi.nlm.nih.gov/books/NBK1311/.

53. Lustbader ED, Williams WR, Bondy ML, Strom S, Strong LC. Segregation analysis in cancer of families of childhood soft-tissue-sarcoma patients. *Am J Hum Genet.* 1992;51(2):344–356.

54. Ognjanovic S, Olivier M, Bergemann T, Hainaut P. Sarcomas in TP53 germline mutation carriers. *Cancer.* 2011;118(5):1387–1396. http://dx.doi.org/10.1002/cncr.26390.

55. Olivier M, Goldgar DE, Sodha N, et al. Li-Fraumeni and related syndromes: correlation between tumor type, family structure, and TP53 genotype. *Cancer Res.* 2003;63(20):6643–6650.

56. Hisada M, Garber J, Li F, Fung C, Fraumeni J. Multiple primary cancers in families with Li-Fraumeni syndrome. *J Natl Cancer Inst.* 1998;90(8):606–611. http://dx.doi.org/10.1093/jnci/90.8.606.

57. Malkin D. Li-Fraumeni syndrome. *Genes Cancer.* 2011;2(4):475–484. http://dx.doi.org/10.1177/1947601911413466.

58. Gonzalez K, Buzin C, Noltner K, et al. High frequency of de novo mutations in Li-Fraumeni syndrome. *J Med Genet.* 2009;46(10):689–693. http://dx.doi.org/10.1136/jmg.2008.058958.

59. National Comprehensive Cancer Network. Genetic/familial high-risk assessment: breast and ovarian. *NCCN Clinical Practice Guidelines in Oncology. Version 2;* 2017. www.nccn.org.

60. *OMIM Entry – # 131100-Multiple Endocrine Neoplasia, Type I; MEN1.* Omimorg; 2016. Available at: https://www.omim.org/entry/131100?search=men1&highlight=men1.

61. Brandi M. CONSENSUS: guidelines for diagnosis and therapy of MEN type 1 and type 2. *J Clin Endocrinol Metab.* 2001;86(12):5658–5671. http://dx.doi.org/10.1210/jc.86.12.5658.

62. Thakker R, Newey P, Walls G, et al. Clinical practice guidelines for multiple endocrine neoplasia type 1 (MEN1). *J Clin Endocrinol Metab.* 2012;97(9):2990–3011. http://dx.doi.org/10.1210/jc.2012-1230.

63. del Pozo C, García-Pascual L, Balsells M, et al. Parathyroid carcinoma in multiple endocrine neoplasia type 1. Case report and review of the literature. *Hormones.* 2011;10(4):326–331. http://dx.doi.org/10.14310/horm.2002.1325.

64. Giusti F, Marini F, Brandi ML. Multiple endocrine neoplasia type 1. In: Pagon RA, Adam MP, Ardinger HH, et al., eds. *GeneReviews® [Internet].* Seattle, WA: University of Washington; August 31, 2005. 1993-2016. Available from: https://www.ncbi.nlm.nih.gov/books/NBK1538/.

65. Thomas-Marques L, Murat A, Delemer B, et al. Prospective endoscopic ultrasonographic evaluation of the frequency of nonfunctioning pancreaticoduodenal endocrine tumors in patients with multiple endocrine neoplasia type 1. *Am J Gastroenterol.* 2006;101(2):266–273. http://dx.doi.org/10.1111/j.1572-0241.2006.00367.x.

66. Gatta-Cherifi B, Chabre O, Murat A, et al. Adrenal involvement in MEN1. Analysis of 715 cases from the Groupe d'etude des Tumeurs Endocrines database. *Eur J Endocrinol.* 2011;166(2):269–279. http://dx.doi.org/10.1530/eje-11-0679.

67. Tham E, Grandell U, Lindgren E, Toss G, Skogseid B, Nordenskjöld M. Clinical testing for mutations in the MEN1 gene in Sweden: a report on 200 unrelated cases. *J Clin Endocrinol Metab.* 2007;92(9):3389–3395. http://dx.doi.org/10.1210/jc.2007-0476.

68. Guo Sawicki M. Molecular and genetic mechanisms of tumorigenesis in multiple endocrine neoplasia Type-1. *Mol Endocrinol.* 2001;15(10):1653–1664. http://dx.doi.org/10.1210/mend.15.10.0717.

69. Lemos M, Thakker R. Multiple endocrine neoplasia type 1 (MEN1): analysis of 1336 mutations reported in the first decade following identification of the gene. *Hum Mutat.* 2008;29(1):22–32. http://dx.doi.org/10.1002/humu.20605.

70. *OMIM Entry – # 171400-Multiple Endocrine Neoplasia, Type IIA; MEN2A.* Omimorg; 2016. Available at: https://www.omim.org/entry/171400?search=ret&highlight=ret.

71. Eng C. The relationship between specific RET proto-oncogene mutations and disease phenotype in multiple endocrine neoplasia type 2. International RET mutation consortium analysis. *JAMA.* 1996;276(19):1575–1579. http://dx.doi.org/10.1001/jama.276.19.1575.

72. Kloos R, Eng C, Evans D, et al. Medullary thyroid cancer: management guidelines of the American thyroid association. *Thyroid*. 2009;19(6):565–612. http://dx.doi.org/10.1089/thy.2008.0403.

73. Marquard J, Eng C. Multiple endocrine neoplasia type 2. In: Pagon RA, Adam MP, Ardinger HH, et al., eds. *GeneReviews® [Internet]*. Seattle, WA: University of Washington; September 27, 1999. 1993-2016. Available from: https://www.ncbi.nlm.nih.gov/books/NBK1257/.

74. Kouvaraki M, Shapiro S, Perrier N, et al. RET protooncogene: a review and update of genotype–phenotype correlations in hereditary medullary thyroid cancer and associated endocrine tumors. *Thyroid*. 2005;15(6):531–544. http://dx.doi.org/10.1089/thy.2005.15.531.

75. Hansford J. Multiple endocrine neoplasia type 2 and RET: from neoplasia to neurogenesis. *J Med Genet*. 2000;37(11):817–827. http://dx.doi.org/10.1136/jmg.37.11.817.

76. Elisei R, Romei C, Cosci B, et al. RET genetic screening in patients with medullary thyroid cancer and their relatives: experience with 807 individuals at one center. *J Clin Endocrinol Metab*. 2007;92(12):4725–4729. http://dx.doi.org/10.1210/jc.2007-1005.

77. Evans D. Neurofibromatosis type 2 (NF2): a clinical and molecular review. *Orphanet J Rare Dis*. 2009;4(1):16. http://dx.doi.org/10.1186/1750-1172-4-16.

78. *OMIM Entry – # 101000-Neurofibromatosis, Type II; NF2*. Omimorg; 2016. Available at: https://www.omim.org/entry/101000?search=nf2&highlight=nf2.

79. Ruggieri M, Praticò A, Evans D. Diagnosis, management, and new therapeutic options in childhood neurofibromatosis type 2 and related forms. *Semin Pediatr Neurol*. 2015;22(4):240–258. http://dx.doi.org/10.1016/j.spen.2015.10.008.

80. Kros J, de Greve K, van Tilborg A, et al. NF2 status of meningiomas is associated with tumour localization and histology. *J Pathol*. 2001;194(3):367–372. http://dx.doi.org/10.1002/path.909.

81. Evans D, Birch J, Ramsden R. Paediatric presentation of type 2 neurofibromatosis. *Arch Dis Child*. 1999;81(6):496–499. http://dx.doi.org/10.1136/adc.81.6.496.

82. Sperfeld A. Occurrence and characterization of peripheral nerve involvement in neurofibromatosis type 2. *Brain*. 2002;125(5):996–1004. http://dx.doi.org/10.1093/brain/awf115.

83. Baser M, Friedman J, Joe H, et al. Empirical development of improved diagnostic criteria for neurofibromatosis 2. *Genet Med*. 2011;13(6):576–581. http://dx.doi.org/10.1097/gim.0b013e318211faa9.

84. Evans D. Neurofibromatosis 2 [bilateral acoustic neurofibromatosis, central neurofibromatosis, NF2, neurofibromatosis type II]. *Genet Med*. 2009;11(9):599–610. http://dx.doi.org/10.1097/gim.0b013e3181ac9a27.

85. Evans D, Ramsden R, Shenton A, et al. Mosaicism in neurofibromatosis type 2: an update of risk based on uni/bilaterality of vestibular schwannoma at presentation and sensitive mutation analysis including multiple ligation-dependent probe amplification. *J Med Genet*. 2007;44(7):424–428. http://dx.doi.org/10.1136/jmg.2006.047753.

86. Wallace A, Watson C, Oward E, Evans D, Elles R. Mutation scanning of the NF2 gene: an improved service based on meta-PCR/sequencing, dosage analysis, and loss of heterozygosity analysis. *Genet Test*. 2004;8(4):368–380. http://dx.doi.org/10.1089/gte.2004.8.368.

87. *OMIM Entry – # 175200-Peutz-Jeghers Syndrome; PJS*. Omimorg; 2016. Available at: https://www.omim.org/entry/175200?search=stk11&highlight=stk11.

88. McGarrity TJ, Amos CI, Baker MJ. Peutz-Jeghers Syndrome. In: Pagon RA, Adam MP, Ardinger HH, et al., eds. *GeneReviews® [Internet]*. Seattle, WA: University of Washington; February 23, 2001. 1993-2016. Available from: https://www.ncbi.nlm.nih.gov/books/NBK1266/.

89. Beggs A, Latchford A, Vasen H, et al. Peutz-Jeghers syndrome: a systematic review and recommendations for management. *Gut*. 2010;59(7):975–986. http://dx.doi.org/10.1136/gut.2009.198499.

90. Hinds R, Philp C, Hyer W, Fell J. Complications of childhood Peutz-Jeghers syndrome: implications for pediatric screening. *J Pediatr Gastroenterol Nutr*. 2004;39(2):219–220. http://dx.doi.org/10.1097/00005176-200408000-00027.

91. McGarrity T. Peutz-Jeghers syndrome. *Am J Gastroenterol*. 2000;95(3):596–604. http://dx.doi.org/10.1016/s0002-9270(99)00890-4.

92. Young R. Sex cord-stromal tumors of the ovary and testis: their similarities and differences with consideration of selected problems. *Mod Pathol*. 2005;18:S81–S98. http://dx.doi.org/10.1038/modpathol.3800311.

93. Syngal S, Brand R, Church J, Giardiello F, Hampel H, Burt R. ACG clinical guideline: genetic testing and management of hereditary gastrointestinal cancer syndromes. *Am J Gastroenterol*. 2015;110(2):223–262. http://dx.doi.org/10.1038/ajg.2014.435.

94. van Lier M, Wagner A, Mathus-Vliegen E, Kuipers E, Steyerberg E, van Leerdam M. High cancer risk in Peutz–Jeghers syndrome: a systematic review and surveillance recommendations. *Am J Gastroenterol*. 2010;105(6):1258–1264. http://dx.doi.org/10.1038/ajg.2009.725.

95. *OMIM Entry – # 158350-Cowden Syndrome 1; CWS1*. Omimorg; 2016. Available at: https://www.omim.org/entry/158350?search=pten&highlight=pten.

96. Pilarski R, Burt R, Kohlman W, Pho L, Shannon K, Swisher E. Cowden syndrome and the PTEN hamartoma tumor syndrome: systematic review and revised diagnostic criteria. *J Natl Cancer Inst*. 2013;105(21):1607–1616. http://dx.doi.org/10.1093/jnci/djt277.

97. Genomic Medicine Institute. *Risk Calculator for Estimation of PTEN Mutation Probability*. Lernerccforg; 2016. Available at: http://www.lerner.ccf.org/gmi/ccscore/.

98. Tan M, Mester J, Ngeow J, Rybicki L, Orloff M, Eng C. Lifetime cancer risks in individuals with germline PTEN mutations. *Clin Cancer Res*. 2012;18(2):400–407. http://dx.doi.org/10.1158/1078-0432.ccr-11-2283.

99. Gorlin R, Cohen M, Condon L, Burke B. Bannayan-Riley-Ruvalcaba syndrome. *Am J Med Genet*. 1992;44(3):307–314. http://dx.doi.org/10.1002/ajmg.1320440309.

100. Zbuk K, Eng C. Cancer phenomics: RET and PTEN as illustrative models. *Nat Rev Cancer.* 2006;7(1):35–45. http://dx.doi.org/10.1038/nrc2037.

101. Eng C. PTEN hamartoma tumor syndrome. In: Pagon RA, Adam MP, Ardinger HH, et al., eds. *GeneReviews® [Internet].* Seattle, WA: University of Washington; November 29, 2001. 1993-2016. Available from: https://www.ncbi.nlm.nih.gov/books/NBK1488/.

102. Bennett KL, Mester J, Eng C. Germline epigenetic regulation of KILLIN in Cowden and Cowden-like syndromes. *J Am Med Assoc.* 2010;304(24):2724–2731.

103. Ni Y, He X, Chen J, et al. Germline SDHx variants modify breast and thyroid cancer risks in Cowden and Cowden-like syndrome via FAD/NAD-dependant destabilization of p53. *Hum Mol Genet.* 2011;21(2):300–310. http://dx.doi.org/10.1093/hmg/ddr459.

104. Orloff M, He X, Peterson C, et al. Germline PIK3CA and AKT1 mutations in Cowden and Cowden-like syndromes. *Am J Hum Genet.* 2013;92(1):76–80. http://dx.doi.org/10.1016/j.ajhg.2012.10.021.

105. Yehia L, Niazi F, Ni Y, et al. Germline heterozygous variants in SEC23B are associated with Cowden syndrome and enriched in apparently sporadic thyroid cancer. *Am J Hum Genet.* 2015;97(5):661–676. http://dx.doi.org/10.1016/j.ajhg.2015.10.001.

106. Eaton K, Tooke L, Wainwright L, Judkins A, Biegel J. Spectrum of SMARCB1/INI1 mutations in familial and sporadic rhabdoid tumors. *Pediatr Blood Cancer.* 2010;56(1):7–15. http://dx.doi.org/10.1002/pbc.22831.

107. *OMIM Entry – # 609322-Rhabdoid Tumor Predisposition Syndrome 1; RTPS1.* Omimorg; 2016. Available at: https://www.omim.org/entry/609322.

108. Swensen J, Keyser J, Coffin C, Biegel J, Viskochil D, Williams M. Familial occurrence of schwannomas and malignant rhabdoid tumour associated with a duplication in SMARCB1. *J Med Genet.* 2008;46(1):68–72. http://dx.doi.org/10.1136/jmg.2008.060152.

109. Schneppenheim R, Frühwald M, Gesk S, et al. Germline nonsense mutation and somatic inactivation of SMARCA4/BRG1 in a family with rhabdoid tumor predisposition syndrome. *Am J Hum Genet.* 2010;86(2):279–284. http://dx.doi.org/10.1016/j.ajhg.2010.01.013.

110. *OMIM Entry – * 608537-VHL Gene; VHL.* Omimorg; 2016. Available at: https://www.omim.org/entry/608537?search=VHL&highlight=vhl.

111. Lonser R, Glenn G, Walther M, et al. Von Hippel-Lindau disease. *Lancet.* 2003;361(9374):2059–2067. http://dx.doi.org/10.1016/s0140-6736(03)13643-4.

112. Frantzen C, Klasson TD, Links TP, et al. Von Hippel-Lindau syndrome. In: Pagon RA, Adam MP, Ardinger HH, et al., eds. *GeneReviews® [Internet].* Seattle, WA: University of Washington; May 17, 2000. 1993-2016. Available from: https://www.ncbi.nlm.nih.gov/books/NBK1463/.

113. Maher E, Neumann H, Richard S. Von Hippel–Lindau disease: a clinical and scientific review. *Eur J Hum Genet.* 2011;19(6):617–623. http://dx.doi.org/10.1038/ejhg.2010.175.

114. Webster A. Clinical characteristics of ocular angiomatosis in von Hippel-Lindau disease and correlation with germline mutation. *Arch Ophthalmol.* 1999;117(3):371. http://dx.doi.org/10.1001/archopht.117.3.371.

115. Kim H, Butman J, Brewer C, et al. Tumors of the endolymphatic sac in patients with von Hippel—Lindau disease: implications for their natural history, diagnosis, and treatment. *J Neurosurg.* 2005;102(3):503–512. http://dx.doi.org/10.3171/jns.2005.102.3.0503.

116. Stolle C, Glenn G, Zbar B, et al. Improved detection of germline mutations in the von Hippel-Lindau disease tumor suppressor gene. *Hum Mutat.* 1998;12(6):417–423. http://dx.doi.org/10.1002/(sici)1098-1004(1998)12:6<417::aid-humu8>3.0.co;2-k.

117. Maher ER, Iselius L, Yates JR, et al. Von Hippel-Lindau disease: a genetic study. *J Med Genet.* 1991;28(7):443–447.

118. VHL Alliance. *Suggested Surveillance.* VHL Alliance; 2016. Available at: https://vhl.org/wp-content/uploads/2016/05/Surveillance-guidelines.pdf.

# CHAPTER 8

# Ethical and Legal Issues

NATHANIEL H. ROBIN, MD • MEAGAN B. FARMER, MS, CGC

## INTRODUCTION

As we have seen in previous chapters, genetic advances have promised many benefits to individuals affected by or at increased risk for cancer. We are entering an era in which we expect genetic testing to allow for the customization of patient care in unprecedented ways. This is the central premise of personalized medicine. However, the expansion of the use of genetic testing has been accompanied by a number of bioethical concerns. Many are similar to the issues we face in all medical testing and are not specific to genetics, whereas some are unique to genetics. All, however, merit careful consideration in the context of genetic testing. This chapter will provide a brief overview of the principles of bioethics, focusing on how they are applied in the setting of genetic evaluation and testing of individuals with a known or suspected cancer predisposition syndrome. In doing so, we will offer an ethical framework with which to approach the ethical dilemmas that may be encountered in the course of clinical practice.

## BIOETHICAL PRINCIPLES

Most healthcare providers have been exposed to the core bioethical principles that are considered the cornerstones of modern bioethics: autonomy, beneficence, nonmaleficence, and justice. It is the balance between these principles that is always in question when one is confronted by an ethically challenging situation in cancer genetic testing. It is therefore essential to understand what each represents.

*Autonomy* refers to the notion of patient self-governance, meaning patients (or in the case of minors, their parents or legal guardians) have the right to make medical decisions independently, based on their own beliefs, and without coercion. Patient autonomy is an overriding principle in modern medicine and is especially valued in western cultures. The notion of the supremacy of patient autonomy was embraced in the 1960s as the concept of paternalism[a] in medicine was increasingly rejected.[1] According to the National Society of Genetic Counselors Code of Ethics,[2] patient autonomy is encouraged when providers allow patients to "make informed independent decisions, free of coercion, by providing or illuminating the necessary facts and clarifying the alternatives and anticipated consequences." In the setting of genetic testing, patient autonomy is achieved through the informed consent process. In a cancer genetics setting, this includes educating the patient on the cancer predisposition condition(s) included in the differential as well as the potential approaches to and benefits, risks, and limitations of genetic testing options. These benefits and risks should be discussed as they apply to both the patient and his/her family, given the implications for the family in a genetics setting.

*Beneficence* refers to the duty of all healthcare providers to aid patients by considering their best medical interests. This involves the healthcare provider taking positive actions to actively do good and prevent harm. It is at the core of patient advocacy. Put another way, beneficence mandates that healthcare providers be motivated by patient best interest rather than other, less noble motives (e.g., reimbursement). In some situations, beneficence and autonomy may be at odds, thereby producing an ethical dilemma. For instance, a provider may offer a medically beneficial genetic test only to have a patient decline this test for herself or her child.

*Nonmaleficence* at its simplest is the concept of doing no harm. It is at the core of the Hippocratic Oath and prohibits injuring the patient through commission or omission. It is important to recognize that some harm may be unavoidable in the setting of genetic testing. For instance, performing predictive testing that may identify that a child is at increased risk for cancer may

---

[a] Paternalism—A philosophy that certain health decisions (e.g., whether to undergo heroic surgery, appropriateness of care in terminally ill patients) are best left in the hands of those providing healthcare. See Arato v. Avedon.

cause psychologic harm to parents, the child, and/or other family members by producing anxiety or in some cases, false reassurance. A practical way to consider nonmaleficence in a clinical setting is to allow harm only when it is unavoidable and/or outweighed by the corresponding benefit in the action. (For example, predictive genetic testing may allow for increased cancer surveillance or risk-reducing measures. However, it may produce anxiety and diminish the autonomy of at-risk relatives.) Like many situations in bioethics, this is often a subjective measure and difficult to determine in an actual clinical setting.

*Justice* refers to the concept of fairness in medicine, meaning the benefits and burdens of healthcare should be distributed equally. At an individual level, this suggests that each person should be entitled to equal medical care, regardless of factors such as ethnic background, geographic location, or ability to pay. It is a lofty goal and is impossible to achieve in practice for every patient. This is also challenging on a societal level, given that healthcare is a finite and, at times, scarce resource. This can be especially challenging in the setting of genetic testing because genetic testing is relatively expensive, and many patients do not have access to clinicians with genetics expertise.

For further information regarding the principles of bioethics, including case examples, see http://depts.washington.edu/bioethx/tools/princpl.html#prin4.[3]

## RIGHT TO KNOW/DUTY TO KNOW

In the context of genetic testing, the *right to know* is most simply defined as the right to know one's genetic status. It is rooted in the principle of autonomy. In a cancer genetics setting, a right to know one's genetic status often means the right to know if one carries a genetic mutation that is associated with a significantly increased risk for cancer, and therefore that one may benefit from advanced cancer surveillance and/or risk-reducing options. Although this concept is fairly straightforward in the context of adult medicine, it can be less straightforward in the pediatric cancer genetics setting. For children with or at increased risk for cancer, who has the right to know? Is it the child's right to know, to the depth that is possible, given that he or she is the one that may be at increased risk and that may benefit from intervention? Is it the parents' right to know this information about their child? Discussions of genetics inherently involve families and balance beneficence, nonmaleficence, and autonomy. Given the limitations of the child to understand the implications

of genetic test results, it could be argued that it is the parents'/guardians' right to know. Some would go a step further and argue that there is a *duty* for parents to know this information about children, especially when there are potential medical benefits for their child. A counterargument is that such actions diminish the child's and other family members' autonomy and their right not to know.

## RIGHT NOT TO KNOW

In contrast to the right to know, but also rooted in autonomy, is the *right not to know* one's genetic status. In many cases, it is the right to avoid the potential psychologic consequences of learning one's genetic status. The early ethics and genetics literature on this subject focused on predictive testing for conditions for which there may be limited options for medical intervention, such as Huntington's disease or Alzheimer's disease. The right not to know may seem less intuitive in a cancer genetics setting because there are often options for medical intervention and screening protocols that reduce the risk for adverse outcomes. However, like most discussions of bioethics, it is not simple or straightforward. These actions may not prevent all adverse outcomes and may certainly create psychologic distress. The nuances of genetic testing in a pediatric setting, including the right not to know, are discussed in more detail in an upcoming section, but the notion does bring up very challenging questions. For instance, do parents have a right not to know about the genetic status of their child in a pediatric cancer genetic setting in which there may be options for medical intervention? Most would agree that this scenario is much different than that of an individual that is considering presymptomatic testing for Huntington's disease or Alzheimer's disease. In the first situation, knowledge of a child's genetic status may allow for interventions that result in earlier detection of cancer or in the reduction of cancer risk. In the latter situations, the potential medical benefits of knowing one's genetic status are minimal. The balance between medical benefit and psychologic harm tilts considerably when weighing these scenarios against one another, demonstrating that the right not to know is often approached differently in a cancer genetics setting than it was in earlier literature on the subject.

## DUTY TO WARN

The *duty to warn* refers to the responsibility of a clinician and/or a patient to disclose genetic information to at-risk individuals. It is rooted in beneficence but may be at odds with autonomy and confidentiality in some scenarios. For a patient deciding whether to disclose genetic information to an at-risk relative, the question of responsibility is an ethical one. For a clinician deciding on whether to disclose genetic information to someone that is not his/her patient, the question of responsibility may also be a legal one.

If a clinician discloses a patient's genetic information to an at-risk relative against his/her patient's wishes, that action breaches confidentiality and therefore the implicit and explicit physician-patient contract. Although one may assume that such an important issue has been thoroughly reviewed at the legal level, there are in fact only two cases that represent legal precedent. In Pate v. Threlkel,[4] Ms. Pate was diagnosed with medullary thyroid carcinoma 3 years after her mother was treated for the same disease. She sued her mother's physician, citing a duty to warn. The court found that the physician had a duty to warn his patient of the familial implications of the disease, but not a duty to breach confidentiality and warn at-risk relatives directly.

However, duty to maintain confidentiality is not absolute in medicine. Consider cases of suspected abuse, gunshot wounds, or times when a patient is deemed an immediate threat to him/herself or society. There is a duty to disclose in these cases. In Safer v. Estate of Pack (1996), Ms. Safer sued her father's physician for failing to warn her that her father died of colon cancer secondary to familial adenomatous polyposis, a condition causing severe polyposis and virtually 100% risk of colorectal cancer without intervention.[5] The court upheld a duty to warn at-risk relatives of the avoidable harm from genetic disease.

In two survey-based studies,[6,7] it was found for both medical geneticists and genetic counselors that it is rare to be faced with the consideration of disclosure without consent, and in those cases, it was uncommon for the genetics professional to actually disclose. Therefore, although this is an important concept to acknowledge and understand, it is fortunately rarely encountered in clinical practice.

In summary, there is considerable uncertainty regarding the duty to warn from a legal precedence standpoint and in the opinions of medical societies. At minimum, clinicians are obliged to inform patients about potential risks to family members. In a pediatric cancer setting, this may mean the patient's parents, siblings and/or future siblings, and extended relatives.

## GENETIC EXCEPTIONALISM

Genetic exceptionalism is the notion that genetic information is somehow different from other medical information. The term was first coined by bioethicist Thomas Murray in Mark A. Rothstein's 1997 book *Genetic Secrets: Protecting Privacy and Confidentiality in the Genetic Era.*[8] Dr. Murray suggested that because genetic information has so many unique features, it must be dealt with in a special manner. However, others have argued that the distinction is invalid and that creating such a special distinction for genetic information is in fact harmful. We will outline the arguments for and against genetic exceptionalism below.

*Genetic information is a predictive diary.* Genetic test results can be used to make predictions about future health and may be used in the diagnosis of a condition before the appearance of symptoms. For instance, if a child is found to have a RET mutation that is causative of multiple endocrine neoplasia type 2A, there is a 95% risk that the child will develop medullary thyroid cancer without intervention, perhaps even in childhood.[9] This may make genetic information seem like a crystal ball through which a child's medical future can be seen. However, although this may feel different than other medical information, this characteristic is not limited to genetic testing. Consider HIV testing, which is used to predict the development of AIDS and a biopsy that demonstrates that a lesion is precancerous. Both are predictive tests that can see (to a limited degree) into an individual's medical future.

*Genetic test results divulge information about other people,* namely, family members. It is true that, when testing a patient for a genetic condition, the family that shares genetic information with the patient is also (in a way) being tested. Because of this, a genetic diagnosis can identify other people (biologic relatives) who are at risk, with more closely related individuals being at greater risk. However, nongenetic tests can also have implications for other people. A positive HIV test has implications for a patient's sex partners. A positive test for tuberculosis has implications for that individual's close contacts, not limited to their biologic relatives. Genetic testing is therefore not the only testing that can have implications for other people; it is the biologic nature of the relationship with at-risk individuals that differs.

*Genetic information has been used to discriminate and to stigmatize.* Genetic information in many forms has been used to discriminate and stigmatize. Although this may seem new to genetic testing, this was the case long before the discovery of the double helix and advent of genetic testing. People (usually those in power and/or in majority) have tried to correlate various traits with genetic inferiority, such as skin color, ethnicity, or cultural identification. There are many examples of discrimination against those with disabilities and/or physical or cognitive differences. Genetically determined traits, such as deafness, small size, and intellectual disability, have all been the subject of discrimination. Furthermore, genetic information is not the only type of medical information that can be or has been used to discriminate. For instance, HIV status, drug and alcohol history, cholesterol and blood pressure measurements, and weight status/body mass index can be used by health insurers to set rates or even deny coverage.

Studies have shown that fear of genetic discrimination is a common concern of patients/parents considering genetic testing. The Genetic Information Nondiscrimination Act (GINA) of 2008 has mitigated much of the risks of discrimination by establishing legal barriers, but the protection is not absolute.[10] GINA and other related legal protections are discussed more completely in the Legal Protection of Genetic Information section.

*Uncovering genetic risk may cause serious psychologic harm.* Learning that you and/or your child has a mutation that markedly increases risk to develop cancer can cause a spectrum of emotions. Many people go through the stages of grief and/or potentially develop anxiety or depression. For this reason, genetic counselors are trained to provide anticipatory guidance and short-term psychosocial counseling to patients and their families and to know when a patient may benefit from referral to a mental health specialist. This is covered in more detail in Chapters 3 and 9, but it is important to realize that these issues also have a bioethics component. Furthermore, while these psychosocial concerns are obviously valid, the fact that they may create anxiety and depression is not unique to genetic testing. Consider a teenager with chronic headaches about to undergo MRI for a suspected brain tumor or an infant with a heart murmur about to undergo echocardiogram for a suspected congenital heart defect. Both are common nongenetic medical tests, and each is considerably anxiety provoking in the parents of the children being tested.

At this point, it should be evident that, although genetic testing does raise many ethical concerns, these may be neither entirely novel nor unique to genetics. Rather, similar concerns accompany other medical tests, and other medical specialties face similar concerns on a regular basis. One difference may be that genetic testing is a relatively new modality using different technology and yielding results in an unfamiliar

language. The "special" aspects of genetic information may seem special in part because they have not been encountered before by many healthcare providers.

Lastly, it is important to note that the idea of genetic exceptionalism is considered by some to not only be inaccurate but also, in fact, harmful in certain instances. By implying that genetic information is so special that it must be approached in an entirely different way than other medical information, we may give genetic information a magical aura that it does not deserve. This can generate both fear and unreasonable expectations among not only the general public but also clinicians, limiting uptake of an important new technology that has tremendous potential benefits for patients and their families.

## LEGAL PROTECTION OF GENETIC INFORMATION

Concerns about insurance discrimination are commonly cited in surveys of both the lay public and medical professionals as risks of undergoing genetic testing. Such concerns may be exaggerated given that there have been few reports of attempts to discriminate using genetic information, and there are existing laws that provide significant protection against abuse to individuals undergoing genetic testing. A discussion of the protections provided by these laws as well as their limitations is included below.

The Health Insurance Portability and Accountability Act (HIPPA; 1996) was created to improve the efficiency and effectiveness of the healthcare system. It set national standards for health identification and security and offers protection against the discrimination of employees and their families based on health factors, such as preexisting medical conditions.[11] The Patient Protection and Affordable Care Act (PPACA) was signed into law by President Barack Obama in 2010. It aimed to expand coverage, increase accountability for health insurance companies, lower healthcare costs, and allow more choices for healthcare consumers. The PPACA strengthens the protection offered by HIPPA as it prohibits group health plans from denying insurance or setting premiums based on preexisting conditions.[12] As we prepare this book for publication, the nation awaits a political shift because Donald Trump recently took President Barack Obama's place in the oval office. Time will tell if this shift impacts the PPACA and the protections it offers.

The GINA may be the most important legislation protecting individuals from discrimination based on genetic information. Signed in to law by President

George HW Bush in 2008 after a decade long series of legislative debates, GINA specifically precludes health insurance companies and employers from using genetic information to determine eligibility for insurance or to set insurance premiums.[10] Genetic information may include genetic test results, the test results of family members, or having a family history of a genetic condition.[10] Employers may not terminate, avoid hiring, or discriminate against any employee based on genetic information.[10] Although GINA significantly bolstered the legal protection of genetic information, it does have limitations. It does not apply to members of the US military, veterans receiving care through Veteran's Administration, or the Indian Health Service.[10]

Although not without limitations, legislation protecting against discrimination based on genetic information has steadily evolved. More work in this area will be crucial as genetic test offerings increase and more providers and patients are aware of its availability. It is important that providers that offer genetic testing to patients be able to address questions or concerns about genetic discrimination or to direct their patients to someone who can, such as a genetic counselor.

## THE SPECIAL SITUATION OF GENETIC TESTING OF CHILDREN

Although much of what has been discussed so far in this chapter pertains to patients of all ages and their families, genetic testing in a pediatric setting introduces a unique set of ethical issues.[13] When an adult elects to proceed with testing for hereditary cancer susceptibility, he or she has usually made an informed decision after weighing the potential benefits (e.g., after a positive test: earlier and more aggressive cancer screening, chemoprevention, prophylactic surgery) and risks (e.g., psychologic distress, concern for life insurance discrimination). An adult in this situation foregoes his or her *right not to know* for his or her *right to know*. This is different in a pediatric setting, as the decision is being made by someone else (parent/guardian) for the patient (minor child). A minor is unable to weigh these risks and benefits. A child's parents are placed in the position to decide whether or not to learn genetic information about their child, which essentially eliminates that child's future right not to know.

Because the vast majority of hereditary cancer susceptibility syndromes do not present in childhood, most bioethicists and genetics professionals believe genetic testing should be delayed until adulthood. If a hereditary cancer syndrome with adult-onset has been identified or is suspected in a family, respect for a child's autonomy and future right not to know override any other concerns given that a diagnosis would not impact the child's medical management until adulthood. This is different than most genetic testing performed in childhood, where the testing is conducted to make a diagnosis.

In a situation where there is concern for a hereditary cancer syndrome with childhood onset, there is a clear benefit to the child as a genetic diagnosis may affect cancer treatment, cancer surveillance, or potentially allow consideration for cancer risk-reducing measures. A genetic diagnosis may also have important implications for adult and minor relatives of the child. If a child has a family history of a hereditary cancer susceptibility syndrome that presents in childhood and he or she tests negative, unnecessary intervention can be avoided. For examples of hereditary cancer syndromes with the potential of manifestation in childhood, see Chapter 6.

See Table 8.1 for additional potential benefits and harms of genetic testing of children.[7] The benefits of multidisciplinary care in a pediatric cancer setting, including mental health support for families making difficult decisions including, but not limited to, genetic testing, are discussed in Chapter 9.

## BIOETHICAL REASONING

Many healthcare professionals know about the field of bioethics, but they have a mistaken understanding of its function and process. They view bioethics as an academic discipline with little practical clinical value and view bioethical reasoning as a subjective exercise with no correct answers for a given situation. This is simply not accurate. Every academic medical center has an ethics committee and an ethics consultation service that is called on to assist in the most difficult clinical situations.

It is important to recognize that clinical bioethics is by definition a field that requires conflict over a clinical question. If all parties agree on a single course of action for a given clinical situation, then there is no need for a bioethics consultation. Rather, bioethics consultations may become involved when there are two or more opinions for the course of action in a given clinical situation. For example, parents wish to continue chemotherapy for their 14-year-old child with leukemia, whereas the child wishes to discontinue treatments and be allowed to die. The purpose of the bioethics consultation in cases such as this is to identify the course of action that is most supported by the ethical principles outlined earlier in this

**TABLE 8.1**
**Potential Benefits and Risks of Genetic Testing in a Pediatric Setting[14]**

| Category | Benefits | Risks |
|---|---|---|
| Medical | Diagnosis confirmation/clarification<br>Increased surveillance<br>Avoidance of needless surveillance/risk-reducing measures | Ineffective, invasive, and/or harmful interventions |
| Reproductive | Ability to plan for birth of child with genetic condition<br>Ability to avoid birth of child with genetic condition | |
| Psychosocial | Potential to psychologically adjust to genetic status<br>Decrease in anxiety/uncertainty<br>Increased ability to make long-term plans (e.g., education, insurance, relationships)<br>Opportunity to alert at-risk family members of genetic risk | Negative impact on self-esteem/self-image<br>Increased anxiety/guilt<br>Alteration of parents' perceptions of child<br>Changed expectations of self/changes in others' expectations<br>Positive genetic test result in family member after disease expression (e.g., after cancer diagnosis)<br>Discrimination concerns (e.g., employment, insurance)<br>Coerced decisions<br>Discovery of nonpaternity/adoption<br>Coerced decision-making |

From American Society of Human Genetics Board of Directors, American College of Medical Genetics Board of Directors. Points to consider: ethical, legal, and psychosocial implications of genetic testing in children and adolescents. *Am J Hum Genet*. 1995;57(5):1233–1241.

chapter. This is done by approaching the case in a systematic, stepwise manner:

1. Define the conflict, and identify which ethical principles are at odds.
2. Determine the medical facts and/or assumptions.
3. List the potential options and alternative courses of action.
4. Evaluate how well each possible course of action is supported by ethical principles.

By following such a systematic approach, one can often arrive at a conclusion that one course of action is the most ethically sound. However, it is important to realize that arriving at an "ethical" decision is not synonymous with deciding the outcome of that case. There are often other factors that must be addressed, such as legal considerations or existing hospital policies. These may and often do conflict with the "ethics" of the situation and typically supersede any ethical decision. Regardless, an ethics consultant's opinion will often provide important context and assistance in leading to a final resolution.

## CASE EXAMPLES

### Case 1

You have a 10-year-old patient with a history of adrenocortical carcinoma. She was found to have a pathogenic TP53 mutation, confirming her molecular diagnosis of Li-Fraumeni syndrome. Her mother was recently tested and found not to have this mutation. As the majority of TP53 mutations are inherited, it is very possible that the father carries the same mutation, but he is estranged from the child and her mother.

You discuss the implications of this result with the patient's mother and stepfather, including options for surveillance that are available for children with Li-Fraumeni syndrome. Your patient has no full siblings, but she has two paternal half-brothers. Her mother and stepfather report that they have full custody of your patient and that the relationship with your patient's father is poor. They refuse to inform him of the risk that he and his other children may have Li-Fraumeni syndrome. Should you attempt to contact your patient's father and disclose his daughter's test result?

1. *Define the ethical issues in conflict*: You want to maintain confidentiality and respect your patient's mother's wishes (autonomy). However, you recognize that this genetic information could have important medical implications for your patient's father and her half-siblings. You have a desire to help these paternal relatives (beneficence) and not to harm them through the omission of information (nonmaleficence).

2. *Determine the medical facts and/or assumptions*: Your patient has a TP53 mutation that she did not inherit from her mother, so she may have inherited it from her father. It could have also been de novo (new in your patient and not inherited from a parent), given that Li-Fraumeni syndrome occurs as a result of de novo mutation in up to 20% of cases. A positive test result in her father would have implications for his medical management and confirm that her paternal half-siblings are at risk. There are surveillance measures that her father and half-brothers could undergo to detect cancers earlier if they test positive for the mutation found in your patient, and these surveillance measures have been shown to increase survival in Li-Fraumeni syndrome.

3. *List the potential options and alternative courses of action*: You could have an in-depth discussion about the medical implications of this diagnosis for your patient's father and half-siblings and stress the importance of the information for these relatives in hopes that the family will reconsider. You could accept that this genetic information is not yours to disclose, drop the subject, and maintain confidentiality. You could tell the family that you will disclose the information if they do not. Lastly, you could contact the patient's father, disclose the test result, and ask that he does not tell the patient's mother that he has been made aware of the information.

4. *Evaluate how well each possible course of action is supported by ethical principles*: Respecting autonomy and patient-physician confidentiality support not disclosing information to the father against the family's will. The best approach may be to help the family understand how important the information is for paternal relatives so that they may disclose on their own and to make yourself available to paternal relatives after this occurs. Ideally, this discussion would take place before the patient's mother was tested.

## Case 2A

You have a 40-year-old patient that was recently found to have a BRCA1 mutation after being diagnosed with breast cancer at age 39. This means she has a molecular diagnosis of hereditary breast and ovarian cancer (HBOC) syndrome. She understands the implications for her medical management and the implications for at-risk relatives, including that this condition is an adult-onset condition. Medical intervention would be indicated for female relatives who test positive at age 25. She requests that her 8-year-old daughter be tested for the BRCA1 mutation identified in her case. Should you test her daughter for this adult-onset condition?

1. *Define the ethical issues in conflict*: You want to respect your patient's wishes (autonomy) and understand that she may have valid personal reasons to want her daughter to undergo genetic testing. This information could eventually be helpful for her daughter's medical management (beneficence). However, you realize that this would not affect her daughter's medical care now, and her daughter may choose not to undergo genetic testing if given the choice as an adult (autonomy).

2. *Determine the medical facts and/or assumptions*: A diagnosis of HBOC has clear medical implications, and there are national guidelines for the management of patients with this condition. However, it is an adult-onset condition and the diagnosis of this condition for a child would not affect his or her medical care.

3. *List the potential options and alternative courses of action*: You could test your patient's daughter, but make sure she understands that increased cancer surveillance should not begin until her daughter is 25 if she tests positive. You could test your patient's daughter only if she promises not to tell her daughter about the result until she is 18. You could refuse to test her daughter at this time and have a discussion with your patient about your reasoning.

4. *Evaluate how well each possible course of action is supported by ethical principles*: Testing the patient's daughter now would be a violation of her future autonomy and with no clear medical benefit. Genetic testing in a child under these circumstances is not recommended by most bioethicists, genetics professionals, or medical societies.

## Case 2B

Consider the previous case scenario, unchanged aside from the patient's daughter's age. What if the patient's daughter was 17, also reported that she is very interested in undergoing genetic testing for her mother's mutation, and was relatively mature for her age?

1. *Define the ethical issues in conflict*: You want to respect the wishes of your patient and her daughter (autonomy). You realize that the information could be helpful for your patient's daughter's medical management (beneficence). However, you do not want to cause psychologic harm by testing her before adulthood or by refusing to test her, which could also cause anxiety (nonmaleficence).

2. *Determine the medical facts and/or assumptions*: A diagnosis of HBOC has clear medical implications, and there are national guidelines for the management of patients with this condition. Genetic testing will be available to her universally next year when she turns

18. However, a positive test result in her case would not affect her medical management until she is 25.

3. *List the potential options and alternative courses of action*: You could refuse to test her at this time but encourage her to come back next year when she is 18 and would no longer be a minor. You could refuse to test her at this time and recommend that she wait until she is 25 given that a positive test result would then have a medical impact. You could have an in-depth discussion with your patient and her daughter about the potential benefits and harms of this test, why there are concerns about genetic testing in minors, and offer testing only if you deem the patient is mature enough to handle the information and/or a mental health professional meets with her and feels she is mature enough to handle the information.

4. *Evaluate how well each possible course of action is supported by ethical principles*: Testing the daughter after true informed consent and after determining that she is mature enough to handle the information supports patient autonomy. Deferring testing until age 18 is somewhat arbitrary (assuming there are no concerns that her age would preclude her from insurance coverage, etc.), given that her medical management would not change at age 18 if she were positive, nor would her maturity level be much different. With any young patient, there should be an emphasis on helping them understand the risks and benefits of genetic testing and factors that may influence personal preferences regarding the timing of testing.

## REFERENCES

1. medical paternalism. (n.d.) McGraw-Hill. *Concise Dictionary of Modern Medicine*. 2002. Retrieved from: http://medical-dictionary.thefreedictionary.com/medical+paternalism.

2. Nsgc.org. *National Society of Genetic Counselors: NSGC Code of Ethics*. 2016. Retrieved from: http://nsgc.org/p/cm/ld/fid=12.

3. Depts.washington.edu. *Bioethic Tools: Principles of Bioethics*. 2016. Retrieved from: http://depts.washington.edu/bioethx/tools/princpl.html#prin4.

4. Florida. District Court of Appeal, First District. Pate v. Threlkel. *Wests South Rep*. August 1, 1994;640:183–186. PMID: 12041296.

5. Liang A. The argument against a physician's duty to warn for genetic diseases: the conflicts created by Safer v. Estate of Pack. *J Health Care Law Policy*. 1998;1(2):437–453. PMID: 16281336.

6. Dugan RB, Wiesner GL, Juengst ET, O'Riordan M, Matthews AL, Robin NH. Duty to warn at-risk relatives for genetic disease: genetic counselors' clinical experience. *Am J Med Genet C Semin Med Genet*. 2003;119C(1):27–34. http://dx.doi.org/10.1002/ajmg.c.10005.

7. Falk MJ, Dugan RB, O'Riordan MA, Matthews AL, Robin NH. Medical geneticists' duty to warn at-risk relatives for genetic disease. *Am J Med Genet A*. 2003;120A(3):374–380. http://dx.doi.org/10.1002/ajmg.a.20227.

8. Rothstein M. *Genetic Secrets*. New Haven: Yale University Press; 1997.

9. Marquard J, Eng C. Multiple endocrine neoplasia type 2. In: Pagon RA, Adam MP, Ardinger HH, et al., eds. *GeneReviews® [Internet]*. Seattle, WA: University of Washington; September 27, 1999. 1993-2017. Available from: https://www.ncbi.nlm.nih.gov/books/NBK1257/.

10. Tan MH. Advancing civil rights, the next generation: the Genetic Information Nondiscrimination Act of 2008 and beyond. *Health Matrix Clevel*. Winter 2009;19(1):63–119. PMID: 19459538.

11. HHS.gov. *HIPAA for Professionals*. 2015. Retrieved from: http://www.hhs.gov/hipaa/for-professionals/index.html.

12. HHS.gov. *Read the Law*. 2015. Retrieved from: http://www.hhs.gov/healthcare/about-the-law/read-the-law/index.html.

13. Botkin JR, Belmont JW, Berg JS, et al. Points to consider: ethical, legal, and psychosocial implications of genetic testing in children and adolescents. *Am J Hum Genet*. 2015;97:6–21.

14. American Society of Human Genetics Board of Directors, American College of Medical Genetics Board of Directors. Points to consider: ethical, legal, and psychosocial implications of genetic testing in children and adolescents. *Am J Hum Genet*. 1995;57(5):1233–1241.

# CHAPTER 9

# Multidisciplinary Care of the Pediatric Cancer Patient

ALEXANDRA CUTILLO, MA • JOSEPH H. CHEWNING, MD •
MICHAEL G. HURST, MD • AVI MADAN-SWAIN, PHD

Pediatric malignancies constitute the fourth leading cause of death in children over 1 year of age in the United States and are second only to unintentional injury in those who are 5–9 years of age.[1] Acute leukemia remains the most common cause of cancer in the pediatric (<18 years of age) population overall, and brain tumors as a group represent the most common solid tumors.[2] The incidence rate of pediatric cancers has remained relatively stable over the past decade.[2,3] However, as a result of significant advances in the treatment and management of pediatric cancer, the number of children and adults surviving pediatric cancer has been increasing over the past four decades.[2]

Extensive basic science research, coupled with national pediatric trials, has yielded significant improvement in the cure rates for children with malignancies. It is estimated that there are more than 400,000 adult survivors of pediatric cancer living in the United States.[4] Intensive multimodal therapy, including chemotherapy, radiation therapy, surgery, and, relatively recently, immunotherapy, is required for successful treatment of most pediatric cancers. These therapies are often effective, but induce significant toxicities for pediatric patients, both acute and chronic.

Over the past decade, research efforts have also focused on the subsequent effects or "costs" incurred as a result of the curative oncologic therapies. These effects are physical, emotional, and psychologic and require a multidisciplinary approach to address the needs of these children both during and after the treatment. Not surprisingly, these studies indicate that these children experience a significant increase in morbidity and mortality as they progress to adulthood.[5]

## MEDICAL THERAPIES FOR PEDIATRIC CANCER

To achieve the substantial improvements that have occurred in pediatric oncology over the past decades, advances in multiple therapeutic modalities have been required. These modalities include chemotherapy agents, immunotherapy, radiation therapy, and surgery. To deliver these therapies, as well as manage the significant and frequently severe toxicities that are incurred during treatment, a multidisciplinary approach is required. Many of these disciplines are shown in Table 9.1. This chapter will focus on the medical management of the pediatric oncology patient, with particular emphasis on the psychosocial impact and treatment.

### Chemotherapy

Oncologic chemotherapy for pediatric cancer was first introduced in the 1940s in the United States.[6] Since that time, the number of chemotherapeutic agents has increased dramatically. Chemotherapy medications are grouped into several categories, based on the source and/or the mechanism of action. Some of the more commonly used medications include the alkylating agents, platinum compounds, antitumor antibiotics, antimetabolites, and topoisomerase-affecting medications.[7,8] In general, these medications act to inhibit the growth of malignant-transformed cells by targeting rapidly dividing cells. As a result, acute toxicities are often seen in other normal tissues characterized by rapid cell turnover, such as the gastrointestinal tract and the bone marrow.

Chemotherapy is administered via intravenous, intramuscular, and oral routes. Safe delivery of intravenous chemotherapy usually requires central venous access but can be given through peripheral access when necessary. Pediatric patients typically receive intravenous chemotherapy in the inpatient setting by licensed practitioners; however, recently there has been attention given to administering more chemotherapy in the outpatient setting.[9,10] Intramuscular and oral chemotherapy treatments are typically administered in the outpatient setting.

Identification of novel agents, as well as determining tumor specificity, occurs following a relatively standardized process. Frequently, a novel agent is tested

**TABLE 9.1**

**Multidisciplinary Needs for Pediatric Oncology Patients**

| Specialty | Procedures |
|---|---|
| Cardiology | Acute cardiac toxicities<br>Heart failure and other long-term toxicities |
| Endocrinology | Hormone deficiencies<br>Secondary diabetes mellitus<br>Growth deficiency |
| Gastroenterology | Nausea and vomiting<br>Gastric ulcers<br>Management of gastrointestinal infections<br>Graft versus host disease |
| Hematopoietic stem cell transplant | Bone marrow/hematopoietic stem cell transplantation |
| Interdisciplinary family support team | Typically includes psychologist, social worker, child life specialist, teacher, chaplain; may also include art and music therapists. Complete psychosocial assessment and provide support and services from diagnosis onward |
| Infectious disease | Infectious complications in immunocompromised patients |
| Nephrology | Management of kidney injury/failure |
| Neurology | Brain and spinal cord toxicities<br>Management and diagnosis of meningitis and encephalitis |
| Neuropsychiatry | Management of psychologic toxicities<br>Total care for patient and family<br>Maintenance of patient autonomy |
| Oncology | Chemotherapy<br>Treatment complications |
| Ophthalmology | Intraocular tumors<br>Intraocular infections<br>Cataracts |
| Orthopedic surgery | Resection and restoration for bone tumors |
| Otolaryngology | Emergent airway management<br>Epistaxis<br>Management of sinusitis and infectious complications |
| Palliative care | Pain management<br>End-of-life care |
| Pulmonology | Management of respiratory failure<br>Acute and chronic pulmonary toxicities<br>Management and diagnosis of pneumonia |
| Radiation oncology | Local tumor radiation<br>Diffuse radiation (total body irradiation) |
| Rehabilitation | Management of neuropathy, muscle weakness, increase strength, movement, endurance |
| Surgery | Tumor resection<br>Venous access<br>Surgical emergencies |
| Urology | Hemorrhagic cystitis<br>Urolithiasis |

against multiple tumor types in vitro, using a variety of high-throughput methodologies.[11-14] Chemotherapeutic agents that are identified as promising agents are next studied in human trials. Initial studies are called Phase I trials and are designed to identify the toxicities/side effects of medications. These studies are important for determining safe dosing by delineating a maximum tolerated dose of the medication.[15,16] Subsequent Phase II studies are designed in the targeted population of patients to determine if the new agent demonstrates efficacy against the specific malignancy. Phase II studies will also provide additional safety and toxicity information. At the conclusion of these studies, the decision will be made as to whether the agent demonstrates activity against a disease when administered at a safe dose. These trials can frequently be combined rather than performed separately (i.e., Phase I/II trials are quite common), especially in rare diseases, such as pediatric malignancies. By combining studies, medications can safely progress more rapidly to larger trials to help advance the treatment for these children.

Larger studies intended to provide clear evidence of efficacy are termed Phase III studies. These trials are performed in larger numbers of patients and typically compare the potential agent with a known standard treatment.[15,16] If studies demonstrate clear efficacy for this agent, the medication will then be submitted to the U.S. Food and Drug Administration (FDA) for approval as a standard therapy for the disease process.

Active chemotherapeutic agents are often given in combination to pediatric patients. Combination chemotherapy has been utilized since the 1960s to increase the rate of clinical remission, decrease chemoresistance rates, and ultimately improve survival rates.[8,17] Typical combination regimens utilize multiple agents that have a different mechanism of action and frequently inhibit cell growth at different aspects of the cell cycle.[8] By utilizing disparate mechanisms of cell killing, combination chemotherapy regimens are able to increase killing of malignant cells by evading resistance and mechanisms of cell repair.[18] Combination chemotherapy regimens now form the backbone of almost all standard and experimental treatment protocols for pediatric malignancies with the exception of novel drug trials, such as Phase I studies.

Through nationally organized studies, cure rates for children with malignancies have rapidly improved over the past decades. However, newer therapies are required to continue this early progress.

## Immunotherapy

Despite the development of multiple novel chemotherapeutic medications, there remains a significant number of patients with chemotherapy-refractory disease or who experience disease relapse following therapy. Other treatment modalities are required for many of these patients to obtain a cure. Over the past years, immunotherapy has become a standard therapy for some malignancies, both upfront and in the setting of disease relapse after treatment.[19] The designation of immunotherapy includes a number of treatment modalities that augment or replace the host immune system to eradicate cancerous cells. These therapies include monoclonal antibodies, adoptive cellular therapy, vaccine therapies, and various other methodologies. As a group, immunotherapies are designed to either complement classic chemotherapy regimens or act as a rescue for patients who do not respond or relapse following these treatments.

Monoclonal antibodies are targeted therapies designed to induce killing of cancerous cells, either directly or by stimulating the immune system.[20] The first therapeutic monoclonal antibody that achieved FDA approval was rituximab. This antibody is directed against human CD20, an antigen commonly expressed on B cell malignancies, i.e., leukemia and lymphoma.[21,22] After binding to CD20, rituximab inhibits proliferation of the B cells and induces antibody-dependent cell-mediated cytotoxicity.[23] Following early success in adult studies, rituximab demonstrated marked efficacy in the treatment of pediatric leukemia and lymphoma.[24,25]

Monoclonal antibodies can also be used to deliver oncologic therapy directly to a cancerous target. Gemtuzumab ozogamicin (Mylotarg) is a monoclonal antibody to human CD33 that is linked to calicheamicin, an antitumor antibiotic that cleaves double-stranded DNA.[26] Gemtuzumab ozogamicin has been shown to be active in treatment of CD33-expressing pediatric acute myelogenous leukemia.[27] Brentuximab vedotin is a monoclonal antibody to human CD30 that is linked to monomethyl auristatin E, a potent tubulin inhibitor. Early pediatric data indicate promising results for the use of this treatment against CD30-expressing lymphomas.[28] In addition to chemotherapies, monoclonal antibodies can be used to deliver other forms of cancer therapy. Ibritumomab tiuxetan is another antihuman CD20 monoclonal antibody; however, it differs from rituximab because it is linked to a radioisotope, yttrium-90 ($^{90}$Y).[29] Improved outcomes have been achieved using ibritumomab tiuxetan in adults with CD20-expressing lymphomas,[30] and early safety data in children are promising.[31] More recently, the use of bispecific antibodies has emerged as another promising form of immunotherapy.

Antibody immunotherapy for malignancies can act to directly kill cancerous cells, or as a mediator to recruit other immune cells, such as T cells and natural killer (NK) cells. Bispecific antibodies act to recruit and activate immune cells for the killing of malignant cells.[32] These antibodies are produced in multiple forms, and the number of these agents is increasing rapidly. The first bispecific antibody to be FDA approved is blinatumomab. Blinatumomab is a bispecific T-cell engager (BiTE) agent that targets CD19 on leukemia and lymphoma cells and recruits T cells to these cells by binding to CD3.[33] Early results using blinatumomab for treatment of pediatric CD19-expressing leukemia have been encouraging.[34,35]

Tumor antigen-specific adoptive cell therapy represents another rapidly growing form of immunotherapy. Genetically altered T cells containing a modified antigen receptor, targeting an antigen expressed on malignant cells, are being developed to treat hematologic malignancies, as well as solid tumors. Patient-derived T cells are genetically engineered with a chimeric antigen receptor (CAR), which is typically introduced using viral vectors, RNA transfection, or other methodologies (reviewed in Refs. 36,37). CAR T cells are expanded in vitro and then administered to the patient. Following infusion, these CAR T cells are then able to detect antigen-expressing malignant cells and deliver a cytotoxic insult. Successful trials have been performed using CD19-specific CAR T cells for adult and pediatric leukemias.[38,39] Other trials utilizing adoptively transferred modified T cells are underway for hematologic malignancies and solid tumors.[37,40,41]

Adoptive cellular therapy using NK cells is another promising therapy for the treatment of malignancies.[42,43] In addition, trials using tumor vaccines and oncolytic viruses offer the promise of new novel therapies for children with cancer.[44,45]

## Radiation Therapy

Radiation therapy remains an important and often indispensable form of treatment for many pediatric malignancies. Radiation is commonly used in the treatment of pediatric soft tissue, bone, and brain tumors, as well as pediatric acute leukemias.[46] The principal of therapy is to deliver the maximal amount of cytotoxicity to cancerous cells while sparing normal tissues as much as possible. Advances in the field of radiation oncology have focused on this goal through the use of multiple techniques, and these advances are partially responsible for the improvements achieved in pediatric cancer outcomes.

Cancer cell killing with radiation therapy occurs through ionizing radiation, which results in deposition of electrons within affected cells. The electrons subsequently interact with multiple cell processes, disrupting the genetic material of the cell and resulting in an inability to undergo cellular division or perform cellular operations.[47] Importantly, normal cells retain an increased ability to repair radiation-induced damage compared with malignant cells; therefore the combination of focused radiation and normal cell healing ideally results in maximal tumor killing with minimal damage to the normal host tissues.[47]

Radiation therapy is generally delivered by either external beam (photon, proton) or internally (brachytherapy). External beam therapy is the most common delivery method of radiation. Multiple radiation modalities exist, differing by the generation of the treatment field (stereotactic body radiation therapy, intensity modulated radiation therapy, and 3D conformal radiotherapy) and/or the form of radiation delivered (photon, electron, proton, and neutron). All of these therapies aim to deliver high-energy radiation to the tumor while minimizing the exposure to the surrounding tissues. Brachytherapy, on the other hand, involves placing a radiation source into the patient to deliver direct radiation to the tumor site.[46] The aim of this therapy is to deliver continuous (rather than intermediate dosing) radiation to the tumor. This delivery method allows for sustained radiation to cancerous cells (increasing the likelihood of radiation exposure during the mitosis and synthesis phases of the cell cycle) with relatively lower dose rate, allowing normal tissues to repair damage more efficiently. Brachytherapy is more commonly used for pediatric soft tissue and bone sarcomas.[48] Radiosurgery is another treatment modality recently introduced, particularly in adult brain tumors. Although the use in pediatrics has been limited, there are encouraging results in the use of radiosurgery in pediatric patients with various brain tumors (reviewed in Ref. 49).

## Surgery

Surgical excision of malignant pediatric tumors has been a cornerstone of oncologic therapy for decades. Despite the increased availability of newer therapies, surgery retains a critical role in treatment and cure of various forms of pediatric cancer, including sarcomas, neuroblastoma, and brain tumors.[50] Prognosis for pediatric patients with many of these tumors is dependent on the degree of surgical excision that can be obtained.[51,52] In addition, pediatric surgery remains critically important for placement of central venous access and other necessary adjunct devices (e.g., percutaneous gastric tubes) as well as management of surgical emergencies in this frequently immunosuppressed population.

## PSYCHOSOCIAL CARE DELIVERY

Advancements in medical management have resulted in increased focus on ensuring that the child/teen and family receive systematic psychosocial services from diagnosis onward. A child/teen's cancer diagnosis has a ripple effect throughout the family system, leaving no member untouched. The cancer journey includes many transitions/phases (diagnosis, remission, relapse, survivorship or end of life and bereavement), each having its own unique medical and psychosocial challenges that necessitate adjustments and adaptations on the part of the child/teen and his/her family. Research indicates that a majority of the families adapt and cope competently to the extraordinary challenges associated with childhood cancer, but approximately one-quarter to one-third of families will experience significant psychosocial difficulties at some point during the course of treatment and will require specific interventions.[53] Regardless, almost all families benefit from some sort of psychosocial support and assistance.

Although there is well-documented literature documenting family strengths and weaknesses in dealing with their child/teen's cancer diagnosis, there is great variability in how these difficulties are assessed and how/which interventions are provided. The child/teen's adjustment to the cancer diagnosis is dependent on his/her individual characteristics and is also influenced by other contextual factors. Some important risk factors include single-parent and/or premorbid strained family relationships, including marital discord, rigid family structure and belief system, financial problems, prior psychiatric history, language barriers, cultural differences, and limited or no family and community support.[54]

To facilitate adaptation and coping, families benefit from ready access to an interdisciplinary (IDT) team of skilled behavioral health professionals, including pediatric psychologist and neuropsychologist, social worker, child life specialists, school teacher, school liaison, chaplain, and expressive therapists (e.g., art and music therapists), over the course of the treatment journey. These family support team members are specifically assigned by the cancer center to work as an IDT family support team or are available through community

consults. Unfortunately, the number of family support team members and how they are organized and accessed vary from one cancer center to the other. This void has resulted in recent efforts to develop pediatric oncology psychosocial care standards for children and their families based on evidence- and consensus-based research.[55] Some of these standards include systematic psychosocial assessment completed by parents (e.g., Psychosocial Assessment Tool) to stratify families by the risk level, as well IDT team members to identify risks and resiliency factors; development of individualized psychosocial care plans that are reviewed frequently by the IDT team and parents to ensure that goals are being addressed; use of evidence-based interventions to address identified difficulties; and continuous close communication between the medical and psychosocial IDT team.[54]

### Phases of Cancer Treatment and Psychosocial Services

Next, we will go through each phase of cancer treatment; identify issues frequently encountered by child/teen, parents, and healthy siblings; and suggest best practice interventions to help maximize child/teen, parents, and healthy sibling adjustment and coping.

#### *Diagnosis and initial treatment*

During the diagnosis and initial treatment phase, families experience a myriad of emotions and feelings ranging from fear, uncertainty, and disruption of family life. They have to become familiar with medical terminology as well as deal with treatment-related demands and side effects. This can be particularly challenging for individuals with limited English proficiency or low education levels.[54] Some common issues experienced during this phase are explained in the following sections.

#### *Managing the shock of diagnosis*

From initiation of medical workup through the formal cancer diagnosis, life begins to change for the child/teen and their family. Parents are typically shocked, are fearful of whether their child/teen will survive, are anxious, and can become increasingly overwhelmed. Both children/teens and parents alike tend to be overwhelmed with feelings of powerlessness and loneliness during this initial phase.[55] Additionally, families may lack information about the psychosocial aspects of childhood cancer. Some *best practice interventions* include the IDT team completing a thorough psychosocial assessment identifying risk and resiliency factors and developing a psychosocial care plan collaboratively.

Particular attention needs to be paid to assessing financial needs, given the documented literature indicating financial difficulties encountered by these families. It is important for the IDT team members to establish trust by listening empathically, and not judging; normalize parents' feelings; prepare parents for possible delay in their own response, as well as possibility that they may cope differently to their child/teen's diagnosis and treatment; stress the importance of taking care of themselves to take care of their child; encourage them to advocate for themselves and their child by asking questions and sharing their concerns (e.g., writing questions on the whiteboard in the hospital room or in a notebook); facilitate referral for baseline neuropsychologic testing if the child/teen's treatment requires central nervous treatment; assist with immediate concrete needs (e.g., transportation, lodging); and provide written information on hospital, local, and national resources.

### Managing disruptions in daily life

The length, intensity, and frequency of outpatient clinic visits and hospitalizations vary by diagnosis and the child/teen's response. Families have to learn how to coordinate medical visits, enforce visitation guidelines so that the child/teen who is immunocompromised is not exposed to infections, manage at-home medication regimens, and deal with physical and emotional treatment-related side effects (e.g., irritability, mood lability, behavioral difficulties, sleep problems, increased appetite secondary to steroids). Additionally, any pre-existing psychosocial difficulties, such as difficulties with concrete needs (e.g., transportation), financial strains, family dynamics, and mental health needs, will likely be exacerbated by the cancer diagnosis and negatively impact family communication, engagement, and medical compliances.[56] Some *best practice interventions* include helping parents identify the needs of all family members and developing strategies to balance competing needs by working closely with the social worker. Particular attention needs to focus on ensuring that arrangements are made for siblings to limit disruptions in their lives. Additionally, the school liaison or hospital teacher can assist the parents with setting up homebound education services for the ill child/teen.

### Communicating about the diagnosis

Many parents struggle with how best to communicate the cancer diagnosis and treatment with child/teen, siblings, and other family members. The child/teen's desire for medical information and engagement in the treatment process is variable and dependent on his/her developmental level.[57,58] Some *best practice interventions*

include encouraging parents to answer questions openly and honestly and provide the child/teen with information at his/her developmental level. This fosters an open, trusting, and supportive relationship among parents, child/teen, and medical and psychosocial team.[59] Additionally, it is helpful for parents to work collaboratively with the child life specialists, who utilize medical play and other tools to explain the diagnosis and medical procedures to the child/teen and healthy sibling. Pediatric psychologists are also skilled in helping the child/teen understand and process the impact of the diagnosis on his/her life. Healthy siblings benefit from coming to the hospital, meeting the medical team and child life specialist, asking questions, and receiving education about their brother/sister's diagnosis and treatment. If this is not possible, the child life specialist can also provide parents with books and other written materials to share with healthy siblings. Ensuring that the child/teen keeps up academically is important. The school liaison or hospital teacher can set up homebound education services for the child/teen unable to attend school. Letters can also be sent to the healthy sibling's teacher, explaining the diagnosis and encouraging monitoring of coping and academic performance. Social workers provide emotional support and assist parents with learning to navigate the medical system, help with employment-related paperwork to provide a job protected leave of absence (i.e., according to the Family and Medical Leave Act of 1993), and provide information about local and national resources. The team chaplain can assist with any spiritual issues that might impact medical care.

### Information and decision-making

Although there is variability in terms of how much information parents seek, with a large percentage expressing a desire for as much information as possible about treatment and prognosis, it is noteworthy that over a third of parents (36%) report finding this information upsetting.[60] For treatment-related decisions, parents tend to rely on their oncologist to help guide the decisions.[60] However, parents are also guided by other sources of information, including the internet, television, friends, and the parents of other patients.[61] Additionally, parents must also navigate nonmedical decisions, such as establishing childcare for the patient and siblings, transportation, and potentially taking a leave of absence from work.

Some *best practice interventions* include careful assessment of parental coping style (e.g., cognitive copers or avoidant), how they process information, and educating parents to view only reliable internet sources of medical information (e.g., CureSearch). For families with limited English proficiency or low education level, information should be presented in small chunks and repeated consistently by all healthcare providers. Additionally, these families benefit from being encouraged to ask questions and, when helpful, from repeating back their understanding of the discussion and plan. As parents begin navigating the medical system, they may benefit from learning problem-solving skills outlined in the Bright Ideas program.[62] This program has been found to decrease negative affectivity in mothers of newly diagnosed patients.[62]

### Dealing with child/teen's physical changes and psychologic reactions

As parents embark on their child's cancer journey, they need to be aware of potential treatment-related side effects (e.g., hair loss, muscle weakness, fatigue). Some *best practice interventions* include encouraging not only parents to be supportive and nurturing but also their child/teen to maintain social interactions and attend school. The child life specialist, pediatric psychologist, and social worker can assist with addressing social withdrawal or anxiety issues related to physical changes and emotional responses. Some children/teens prefer to work through their emotions nonverbally and will benefit from working with an art or music therapist.

### Sibling reactions

Often siblings sense something is wrong because their parents are anxious and may not be aware of the ill child/teen's cancer diagnosis. Sometimes, healthy siblings feel responsible for the ill child/teen's cancer diagnosis (e.g., think they "wished" it because they were angry with them). Changes in household routines contribute to siblings experiencing distress and confusion over what to expect during the treatment course. Some *best practice interventions* include dispelling any myths that they were responsible for cancer diagnosis and encouraging siblings to visit the hospital, meet with the medical and psychosocial IDT teams, and ask questions. Encourage parents to set aside time to engage in special activities with the healthy siblings so that they do not feel abandoned or isolated. Additionally, use of communication channels such as FaceTime and Skype are helpful ways to maintain communication between the well sibling, ill child/teen, and caretaker parents in the hospital.

### Maintaining and accessing social support

Social support plays an important role in the postdiagnosis adjustment process. Some *best practice interventions* include the IDT team carefully assessing available social support and willingness of the parents to reach

out and seek assistance. Encourage parents to make a list of tasks that they need help with and give it to a designated family member or friend who can disseminate it to others. It may help to encourage the family to set up a care team through their church or local community to help with specific needs (e.g., transportation of healthy sibling to extracurricular activity, mowing the yard), with our without the use of a webpage (e.g., CaringBridge), to keep family and friends informed about their child/teen's medical progress.

### Remission

Medical treatments vary in lengths, ranging from months to years, as well as intensity. Although many families adjust to dealing with the chronicity of the treatment course, financial strain and increased parent/caregiver stress and distress emerge. As treatment progresses, many children experience a favorable response, but families are fearful of the possibility of relapse. Additionally, many children and adolescents are isolated from peers during active treatment and unable to attend school because they are immunocompromised and susceptible to infections.[54]

### Adjustment and impact on family

The needs of the sick child are prioritized above those of other family members, and the roles and responsibilities of family members shift to accommodate this change. The ill child/teen continues to be the focus of attention within the family, often leading to feelings of loneliness among healthy siblings. Families are often "split" with one parent managing work and household duties, whereas the other stays with the ill child in the hospital. Although some families report that the family bond forged during treatment makes them stronger after completion of treatment, others report heightened family or marital stress during the active treatment phase.[56,63] Some *best practice interventions* include the IDT team closely monitoring family functioning and updating the psychosocial care plan to reflect changes in concrete needs as well as parent stress/distress and interventions to address these issues. Additionally, parents should be encouraged to take breaks when possible and continue using problem-solving to address any new needs that arise. Adjustment difficulties experienced by the ill child/teen secondary to treatment, including self-esteem, body image, and changes in personal identity, need to be closely monitored. The pediatric psychologist can work with the child/teen experiencing coping difficulties through the use of cognitive behavior therapy or acceptance-based therapy. Additionally, the ill child/teen should attend school when medically able; when cleared to attend school regularly, the school liaison and child life specialist can work with the child/teen to develop a plan to facilitate smooth and successful school reentry. Healthy diet and daily exercise for the child/teen to build strength and endurance should also be a part of the family's daily routine. Physical therapists can prescribe a workout program for the child/teen, and the nutritionist can assist with planning healthy meals.

## Completing Treatment and Survivorship

On completion of medical treatment and during survivorship, parents report experiencing mixed emotions. Additionally, cancer survivors and parents may experience symptoms of posttraumatic stress disorder several years after completion of therapy. Although there is a sense of relief that treatment has ended, there is also fear and concern about potential for relapse and decreased interactions with medical team.[53] Some common issues experienced during this phase are explained in the following sections.

### Ambivalent feelings

As treatment draws to a close, the parents will experience mixed emotions, adjust to treatment late effects, learn to adjust to a "new normal," and understand the need to maintain appropriate medical follow-up care. Some *best practice interventions* include educating family about typical feelings, including uncertainty, ambivalence, and anxiety, experienced by parents and providing community resources to assist with these emotions. Additionally, the ill child/teen may experience similar emotions, have difficulty shifting their perspective from being a "patient" to being a "survivor", and need to be referred to the pediatric psychologist.

### Medical late effects

Both the diagnosis and treatment may result in long-term physical and psychologic sequelae. The child/teen may experience symptoms of posttraumatic stress syndrome and/or learning and academic difficulties. *Best practice interventions* include referring child/teen who received central nervous system treatment as part of their medical therapy for follow-up neuropsychologic evaluations at regular intervals. Additionally, any child/teen experiencing emotional difficulties should be referred to a pediatric psychologist experienced in dealing with survivor issues.

## Disease Recurrence and Death

Despite treatment advances, some children/teens may unfortunately experience disease recurrence, which is emotionally distressing and challenging for all family members. Parents frequently experience shock and disbelief followed by increased symptoms of psychologic distress, anxiety, anger, and depression. This is accompanied by an urgent need to explore the possibility of other curative options, including second opinions. At times, parents cope and communicate differently with each other and struggle with how to share the information with the ill child/teen. During this painful period, the IDT team members who have close working relationships with the family need to be available, acknowledge reactions and feelings, monitor these symptoms, and make additional referrals (e.g., psychiatrist), particularly if the symptoms are severe or reactivate a previous mental illness. If the parent is reluctant to see a professional therapist, it is important to assess for other sources of support and encourage them to share their feelings, fears, and concerns with a trusted friend and/or religious leader. As parents work through their emotions, journaling has been found to be an effective alternative intervention.

Open discussions of treatment options, including obtaining a second opinion from another center, are important. When medically indicated, there should be a shift in focus from "cure" to open discussion about palliation or symptom control. For the child/teen, it is important to provide developmentally appropriate information regarding prognosis. Answer questions honestly while respecting parental wishes/beliefs. When appropriate, the ill child/teen should be engaged in open discussion to make sure their wishes are heard. Additionally, the art therapist can provide opportunities for the family to create a "legacy" piece.

The anticipated and actual death of the child/teen is a painfully intense experience, and family members experience heightened psychologic, physical, behavioral, spiritual, existential, and social distress. Family members are at risk for immediate and long-term difficulties because they deal with the painful experience of losing a child/teen.[54]

More detailed information on dealing with disease recurrence and death is presented next in the palliative and supportive care section.

## ROLE OF PALLIATIVE CARE THROUGHOUT TREATMENT

An unavoidable consequence of malignancy as a leading cause of death in children is the considerable burden caused by suffering, particularly at the end of life. Up to 89% of children experience significant suffering in the last month of life.[64] This comes not only in the form of physical pain but also in the form of emotional, spiritual, and existential distress. Although not all younger children may experience this full spectrum of discomfort, children as young as 7 years can report clinically pertinent and consistent information about symptoms beyond those that are primarily physical. Additionally, parents of children affected by cancer have demonstrated a multidimensional experience of pain, fear, failure, despair, powerlessness, hopelessness, purposelessness, and vulnerability.[65]

Palliative care, with the intent of reduction of suffering and improved care, has a clear role for these patients and their families.[66] The WHO includes palliative care as a part of a comprehensive approach to cancer that "improves the quality of life of patients and their families facing the problems associated with life-threatening illness, through the prevention and relief of suffering by means of early identification and impeccable assessment, and treatment of pain and other problems—physical, psychosocial, and spiritual."[67] Applied to the pediatric population, the American Academy of Pediatrics (AAP) supports an integrated model of palliative care, whereby "the components of palliative care are offered at diagnosis and continued throughout the course of illness, whether the outcome ends in cure or death."[68]

There are four primary categories of disease appropriate for palliative care: (1) diseases for which curative, restorative, or life-extending treatment is possible but may fail; (2) diseases requiring prolonged periods of intensive treatment, with intent at prolonging length and quality of life; (3) progressive conditions, where treatment is primarily palliative; and (4) severe, but nonprogressive, conditions leading to disability with multiple expected sequelae.[69] Cancer falls in the first of these categories, and fortunately, with ~85% 5-year survival in the pediatric population, failure to cure is less common than for many other disease states.[70]

The American Society of Clinical Oncology advises early integration of palliative care and oncology care for all cancer patients with high-risk disease or high symptom burden, based on strong evidence that integration soon after diagnosis improves patient and caregiver outcomes.[71] The AAP's committee on Bioethics and Hospital Care validates that "reserving palliative care for children who have exhausted every curative treatment and are dying would mean that many other children would miss out on the benefits that palliative care can offer" and that "including children who have a life-threatening illness or condition but are still receiving curative treatment ensures that all children who can benefit from palliative care have access to it."[68]

The model for appropriate palliative care involvement (bottom figure) illustrates the presence throughout the disease process, from the time of diagnosis, steadily increasing as/if disease progresses, with maximum involvement as peak symptom burden appears, continuing even after death, and tapering through the bereavement process. The old model (top figure) portrays the original use of hospice and palliative care services, before its evolution into the current, integrated form.[72]

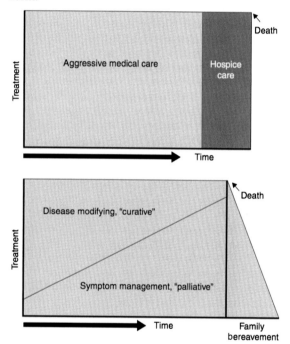

The AAP proffers five primary tenets for palliative care, with respect to the specialty's role in care of children with terminal illness:

1. Respect for dignity of patients and families
2. Access to competent and compassionate palliative care
3. Support for caregivers
4. Improved professional and social support
5. Continued improvement of pediatric palliative care through research and education[68]

Respect for dignity of patients and families comes in several forms, most important being inclusion of patients, when able, in information sharing and decision-making. The role of the palliative care clinician is to elicit goals and values of a family, as they relate specifically to illness, and to offer recommendations for next steps in care, integrating the objective medical data to come to a mutually agreeable treatment decision.

This is in addition to provision of optimal symptom management. There is clearly a great deal of overlap between this responsibility and that of the pediatric oncologist, and the unique perspective of a palliative care team can serve to enhance the care of the patient, working collaboratively with the oncology team.

Access to competent and compassionate palliative care is a major barrier to comprehensive care of children with malignancies. Sixty percent of pediatric oncology centers have no formal palliative care program.[73] This gap is filled to the best extent possible by oncology providers, and yet nearly three-quarters (71%) of oncology fellowship programs are without formal palliative care curriculum.[74] As long as this is the case, it becomes even more vital that the role of the oncologist is focused not only on medical and symptomatic treatments, but also in consideration of the patient and family as a whole. Much of the time, the role of support for caregivers falls appropriately to members of the interdisciplinary team. At many institutions, this team is more closely related to oncology than to palliative care and serves the primary role of support of patients and caregivers.

The palliative care team collectively plays several primary roles, most easily delineated when considering the inpatient setting. The team serves the function of advanced care coordination, enhancing communication across settings, facilitating decision-making with patients and families, and ensuring appropriate access for management of symptoms and support. These duties are essential for maintaining a patient-focused and relationship-centered approach to care.

The team is also involved in ethical issues, many times in conjunction with a dedicated ethics committee, where one exists. Their role in this capacity serves to ensure that all treatment decisions are made in the best interest of the child. This requires shared decision-making with both patients and families, as well as the child's primary oncologist. Palliative providers can assist in making judgments about withholding or withdrawing certain therapies and in supporting parental decision-making authority regarding discontinuation of nonbeneficial therapies.

Adolescents desire autonomy in making choices about the kind of medical treatment they desire, the ways they would like to be cared for, information they want family and friends to have, and how they would like to be remembered.[75] The National Institute of Health's guide, *Voicing My Choices: A Planning Guide for Adolescents and Young Adults*, can be a valuable resource in guiding some of these conversations among families and medical teams. This tool attempts to help families and health professionals open difficult conversations

and was developed using language and questions tailored to the particular needs and preferences of young people. It can also be helpful for the development of identity at a time when this is a typical need and allows for collective thinking about the legacy a young adult may leave behind.[76]

Emotional, psychosocial, and spiritual support are offered in conjunction with the IDT team, which ideally includes a child life therapist, counselor, music therapist, chaplain, and social worker. There is evidence that children search for deeper understanding of their experiences and that the key to emotional coping with serious illness and disability can frequently be found within the realm of spirituality.[77] The IDT partners to provide a holistic assessment and intervention that allows improved coping.

Most acutely, the palliative clinician works to provide symptom control in the physical realm. This includes pain of all types, constipation, anxiety, agitation, delirium, nausea, secretions, and pruritis, among others. Standard symptom control measures are utilized, along with more unorthodox interventions for particularly recalcitrant symptoms. When symptoms are severe, discussion of risks and benefits of aggressive symptom management that may contribute to unwanted side effects is pursued. The ultimate aim is for manageable symptom control, balanced with those potential side effects, with sedation being the primary issue for many symptom medications. Although opioids are of concern to some for their potential for long-term negative effects, evidence suggests that for children who are symptomatic from uncontrolled cancer-related pain, worries of addiction should not be of import. This is not an issue for appropriately utilized for opioids used judiciously in serious illness.[78]

The distinction between palliative care and hospice is an important one to make. Hospice is most accurately described as a very small portion of palliative care, the latter of which should be available at any point during an acute or chronic illness that causes the patient to experience distress in any realm of suffering. It is appropriate for nearly every patient with a chronic or potentially incurable illness. Hospice, conversely, is a primarily comfort-focused approach to care, typically in the home setting, that becomes appropriate only in the last 6 months of an illness. The intent is ongoing palliation, when continued decline is expected.

Outside the hospital setting, there remains a role for both palliative care and hospice. There is apparent value in palliative home care delivered concurrently with oncology care. Compared with oncology care alone, symptom distress experiences were similar, but quality of life was improved, and patients were more likely to die at home, rather than while hospitalized.[79] Similarly, specialist pediatric palliative care services significantly reduced the number of planned hospital admissions for children with cancer, showing potential personal, social, and economic benefits.[80]

As the importance of both quality and quantity of life in terminal illness is well-recognized, especially in the pediatric population, the 2010 Patient Protection and Affordable Care Act allowed for Concurrent Care for Children.[73] Through this provision, palliative and hospice care services must be reimbursed if given to a child who has a life-limiting illness and is eligible for Medicaid or the Children's Health Insurance Program. This holds true even when the child is still receiving disease-modifying treatments, such as chemotherapy. This allows for inclusion of palliative-minded care from diagnosis, with, as disease progresses, increasing focus on identification, prevention, and alleviation of suffering.[74] However, it does not preclude traditional medicine that may add to comfort, including antibiotics, transfusions, and palliative chemotherapy.[81] In this way, palliative and oncology care are integrated by using disease-directed therapy in conjunction with quality of life measures.

In summary, integration of palliative care with oncology care is crucial in the holistic approach to serious illness that addresses disease state, physical, emotional, spiritual, and psychosocial suffering. This is best accomplished via close partnership with the oncologist, palliative care clinician, and IDT that includes a chaplain, psychologist, child life therapist, music therapist, and social worker. Inclusion of all of these parties ensures that a patient and family is enveloped with care that is multifaceted and is as effective as possible at addressing the frequent and significant suffering that exists as a result of serious, chronic, or terminal illness. This is especially true in the realm of genetically predisposed malignancies, given the added complexity of other current or even potential future family members who are at risk for similar conditions and related suffering. That added layer of psychosocial implications certainly makes the case for improved quality of life through the proven efficacy of the palliative and the interdisciplinary team.

## REFERENCES

1. Centers for Disease Control, Prevention. *Injury Prevention & Control: Data & Statistics*; 2016.
2. National Cancer Institute. *Surveillance, Epidemiology, and End Results (SEER) Program*; 2017.
3. Ward E, DeSantis C, Robbins A, Kohler B, Jemal A. Childhood and adolescent cancer statistics. *CA Cancer J Clin.* 2014;2014(64):83–103.
4. Robison LL, Hudson MM. Survivors of childhood and adolescent cancer: life-long risks and responsibilities. *Nat Rev Cancer.* 2014;14:61–70.
5. Bhatia S, Armenian SH, Armstrong GT, et al. Collaborative research in childhood cancer survivorship: the current landscape. *J Clin Oncol.* 2015;33:3055–3064.
6. Farber S, Diamond LK. Temporary remissions in acute leukemia in children produced by folic acid antagonist, 4-aminopteroyl-glutamic acid. *N Engl J Med.* 1948;238:787–793.
7. Sparreboom AEW, Baker SD. Chemotherapy in the pediatric patient. In: Fisher D, Orkin SH, Look TA, Lux SE, Ginsburg D, Nathan DG, eds. *Oncology of Infancy and Childhood.* 1st ed. Philadelphia, PA: Saunders Elsevier; 2009:174–208.
8. Adamson PCBS, Bagatell R, Skolnik JM, Balis FM. General principles of chemotherapy. In: Philip A, Pizzo MD, David G, Poplack MD, eds. *Principles and Practice of Pediatric Oncology.* 7th ed. Philadelphia, PA: Wolters Kluwer; 2016:239–315.
9. Stiff PJ. Managing hematopoietic stem-cell transplant resources: the case for outpatient transplantation. *Leuk Lymphoma.* 2009;50:6–7.
10. Vozniak M, Wiley K, Kucharczuk C, et al. Transitioning chemotherapy administration from the inpatient setting: creating bed capacity and improving the patient experience. *J Clin Oncol.* 2012;30:152.
11. Lecault V, Vaninsberghe M, Sekulovic S, et al. High-throughput analysis of single hematopoietic stem cell proliferation in microfluidic cell culture arrays. *Nat Methods.* 2011;8:581–586.
12. Macarron R, Banks MN, Bojanic D, et al. Impact of high-throughput screening in biomedical research. *Nat Rev Drug Discov.* 2011;10:188–195.
13. Cosson S, Lutolf MP. Hydrogel microfluidics for the patterning of pluripotent stem cells. *Sci Rep.* 2014;4:4462.
14. Das V, Bruzzese F, Konecny P, Iannelli F, Budillon A, Hajduch M. Pathophysiologically relevant in vitro tumor models for drug screening. *Drug Discov Today.* 2015;20:848–855.
15. *Clinical Trials.* 2017. http://www.cancer.net.
16. *Clinical Studies.* 2017. http://www.clinicaltrials.gov.
17. Henderson ES, Samaha RJ. Evidence that drugs in multiple combinations have materially advanced the treatment of human malignancies. *Cancer Res.* 1969;29:2272–2280.
18. Cree IA, Charlton P. Molecular chess? Hallmarks of anticancer drug resistance. *BMC Cancer.* 2017;17:10.
19. Huang MA, Krishnadas DK, Lucas KG. Cellular and antibody based approaches for pediatric cancer immunotherapy. *J Immunol Res.* 2015;2015:1–7.
20. Marabelle A, Gray J. Tumor-targeted and immune-targeted monoclonal antibodies: going from passive to active immunotherapy. *Pediatr Blood Cancer.* 2015;62:1317–1325.

21. Miller RA, Maloney DG, Warnke R, Levy R. Treatment of B-cell lymphoma with monoclonal anti-idiotype antibody. *N Engl J Med.* 1982;306:517–522.

22. Meeker TC, Lowder J, Maloney DG, et al. A clinical trial of anti-idiotype therapy for B cell malignancy. *Blood.* 1985;65:1349–1363.

23. Maloney DG, Grillo-Lopez AJ, White CA, et al. IDEC-C2B8 (Rituximab) anti-CD20 monoclonal antibody therapy in patients with relapsed low-grade non-Hodgkin's lymphoma. *Blood.* 1997;90:2188–2195.

24. Griffin TC, Weitzman S, Weinstein H, et al. A study of rituximab and ifosfamide, carboplatin, and etoposide chemotherapy in children with recurrent/refractory B-cell (CD20+) non-Hodgkin lymphoma and mature B-cell acute lymphoblastic leukemia: a report from the Children's Oncology Group. *Pediatr Blood Cancer.* 2009;52:177–181.

25. Goldman S, Smith L, Anderson JR, et al. Rituximab and FAB/LMB 96 chemotherapy in children with Stage III/IV B-cell non-Hodgkin lymphoma: a Children's Oncology Group report. *Leukemia.* 2013;27:1174–1177.

26. Sievers EL, Larson RA, Stadtmauer EA, et al. Efficacy and safety of gemtuzumab ozogamicin in patients with CD33-positive acute myeloid leukemia in first relapse. *J Clin Oncol.* 2001;19:3244–3254.

27. Pollard JA, Loken M, Gerbing RB, et al. CD33 expression and its association with gemtuzumab ozogamicin response: results from the randomized phase III Children's Oncology Group trial AAML0531. *J Clin Oncol.* 2016;34:747–755.

28. Locatelli F, Neville KA, Rosolen A, et al. Phase 1/2 study of brentuximab vedotin in pediatric patients with relapsed or refractory (R/R) Hodgkin lymphoma (HL) or systemic anaplastic large-cell lymphoma (sALCL): preliminary phase 2 data for brentuximab vedotin 1.8 mg/kg in the HL study arm. *Blood.* 2013;122:4378.

29. Knox SJ, Goris ML, Trisler K, et al. Yttrium-90-labeled anti-CD20 monoclonal antibody therapy of recurrent B-cell lymphoma. *Clin Cancer Res.* 1996;2:457–470.

30. Witzig TE, Gordon LI, Cabanillas F, et al. Randomized controlled trial of yttrium-90-labeled ibritumomab tiuxetan radioimmunotherapy versus rituximab immunotherapy for patients with relapsed or refractory low-grade, follicular, or transformed B-cell non-Hodgkin's lymphoma. *J Clin Oncol.* 2002;20:2453–2463.

31. Cooney-Qualter E, Krailo M, Angiolillo A, et al. A phase I study of 90yttrium-ibritumomab-tiuxetan in children and adolescents with relapsed/refractory CD20-positive non-Hodgkin's lymphoma: a Children's Oncology Group study. *Clin Cancer Res.* 2007;13:5652s–5660s.

32. Thakur A, Lum LG. "NextGen" biologics: bispecific antibodies and emerging clinical results. *Expert Opin Biol Ther.* 2016;16:675–688.

33. Hoffman LM, Gore L. Blinatumomab, a bi-specific anti-CD19/CD3 BiTE((R)) antibody for the treatment of acute lymphoblastic leukemia: perspectives and current pediatric applications. *Front Oncol.* 2014;4:63.

34. Schlegel P, Lang P, Zugmaier G, et al. Pediatric posttransplant relapsed/refractory B-precursor acute lymphoblastic leukemia shows durable remission by therapy with the T-cell engaging bispecific antibody blinatumomab. *Haematologica.* 2014;99:1212–1219.

35. von Stackelberg A, Locatelli F, Zugmaier G, et al. Phase I/Phase II study of blinatumomab in pediatric patients with relapsed/refractory acute lymphoblastic leukemia. *J Clin Oncol.* 2016;34:4381–4389.

36. Maude SL, Teachey DT, Porter DL, Grupp SA. CD19-targeted chimeric antigen receptor T-cell therapy for acute lymphoblastic leukemia. *Blood.* 2015;125:4017–4023.

37. Ye B, Stary CM, Gao Q, et al. Genetically modified t-cell-based adoptive immunotherapy in hematological malignancies. *J Immunol Res.* 2017;2017:5210459.

38. Porter DL, Levine BL, Kalos M, Bagg A, June CH. Chimeric antigen receptor-modified T cells in chronic lymphoid leukemia. *N Engl J Med.* 2011;365:725–733.

39. Maude SL, Frey N, Shaw PA, et al. Chimeric antigen receptor T cells for sustained remissions in leukemia. *N Engl J Med.* 2014;371:1507–1517.

40. Zhang Q, Zhang Z, Peng M, Fu S, Xue Z, Zhang R. CAR-T cell therapy in gastrointestinal tumors and hepatic carcinoma: from bench to bedside. *Oncoimmunology.* 2016;5:e1251539.

41. Yong CS, Dardalhon V, Devaud C, Taylor N, Darcy PK, Kershaw MH. CAR T-cell therapy of solid tumors. *Immunol Cell Biol.* 2017. http://dx.doi.org/10.1038/icb.2016.128.

42. Sinha C, Cunningham LC. An overview of the potential strategies for NK cell-based immunotherapy for acute myeloid leukemia. *Pediatr Blood Cancer.* 2016;63:2078–2085.

43. Venstrom JM, Pittari G, Gooley TA, et al. HLA-C-dependent prevention of leukemia relapse by donor activating KIR2DS1. *N Engl J Med.* 2012;367:805–816.

44. Cripe TP, Chen CY, Denton NL, et al. Pediatric cancer gone viral. Part I: strategies for utilizing oncolytic herpes simplex virus-1 in children. *Mol Ther Oncolytics.* 2015;2.

45. Elster JD, Krishnadas DK, Lucas KG. Dendritic cell vaccines: a review of recent developments and their potential pediatric application. *Hum Vaccin Immunother.* 2016;12:2232–2239.

46. Ermoian RF, Braunstein S, Mishra KM, Kun L, Haas-Kogan DA. General principles of radiation oncology. In: Pizzo PA, Poplack DG, eds. *Principles and Practice of Pediatric Oncology.* 7th ed. Philadelphia, PA: Wolters Kluwer; 2016:362–383.

47. Begg AC, Stewart FA, Vens C. Strategies to improve radiotherapy with targeted drugs. *Nat Rev Cancer.* 2011;11:239–253.

48. Lloyd S, Alektiar KM, Nag S, et al. Intraoperative high-dose-rate brachytherapy: an American Brachytherapy Society consensus report. *Brachytherapy.* 2017;16.

49. Murphy ES, Chao ST, Angelov L, et al. Radiosurgery for pediatric brain tumors. *Pediatr Blood Cancer.* 2016;63:398–405.

50. Dasgupta R, Billmire D, Aldrink JH, Meyers RL. What is new in pediatric surgical oncology? *Curr Opin Pediatr.* 2017;29:3–11.

51. Osasan S, Zhang M, Shen F, Paul PJ, Persad S, Sergi C. Osteogenic sarcoma: a 21st century review. *Anticancer Res.* 2016;36:4391–4398.

52. Massimino M, Giangaspero F, Garre ML, et al. Childhood medulloblastoma. *Crit Rev Oncol Hematol.* 2011;79:65–83.

53. Long KA, Marsland AL. Family adjustment to childhood cancer: a systematic review. *Clin Child Fam Psychol Rev.* 2011;14:57–88.

54. Madan Swain A, Hinds PS. Impact of cancer on family and siblings. In: Wiener LS, Pao M, Kazak AE, Kupst MJ, Patenaude AF, eds. *Pediatric Psycho-Oncology: A Quick Reference on the Psychosocial Dimensions of Cancer Symptom Management.* 2nd ed. Oxford University Press; 2015.

55. Wiener L, Kazak AE, Noll RB, Patenaude AF, Kupst MJ. Standards for the psychosocial care of children with cancer and their families: an introduction to the special issue. *Pediatr Blood Cancer.* 2015;62:419–424.

56. Darcy L, Knutsson S, Huus K, Eskar K. The everyday life of the young child shortly after receiving a cancer diagnosis, from both children's and parent's perspectives. *Cancer Nurs.* 2014;37:445–456.

57. Brand SR, Fasciano K, Mack JW. Communication preferences of pediatric cancer patients: talking about prognosis and their future life. *Support Care Cancer.* 2017;25:769–774.

58. Lambert V, Glacken M, McCarron M. Communication between children and health professionals in a child hospital setting: a child transitional communication model. *J Adv Nurs.* 2011;67:569–582.

59. NIH. *Children with Cancer: A Guide for Parents*; 2015. Available at: https://www.cancer.gov/publications/patient-education/children-with-cancer.pdf.

60. Mack JW, Wolfe J, Grier HE, Cleary PD, Weeks JC. Communication about prognosis between parents and physicians of children with cancer: parent preferences and the impact of prognostic information. *J Clin Oncol.* 2006;24:5265–5270.

61. Kilicarslan-Toruner E, Akgun-Citak E. Information-seeking behaviours and decision-making process of parents of children with cancer. *Eur J Oncol Nurs.* 2013;17:176–183.

62. Sahler OJZ, Dolgin MJ, Phipps S, et al. Specificity of problem-solving skills training in mothers of children newly diagnosed with cancer: results of a multisite randomized clinical trial. *J Clin Oncol.* 2013;31:1329–1335.

63. da Silva FM, Jacob E, Nascimento LC. Impact of childhood cancer on parents' relationships: an integrative review. *J Nurs Scholarsh.* 2010;42:250–261.

64. Wolfe J, Grier HE, Klar N, et al. Symptoms and suffering at the end of life in children with cancer. *N Engl J Med.* 2000;342(5):326–333.

65. Collins JJ, Devine TD, Dick GS, et al. The measurement of symptoms in young children with cancer: the validation of the Memorial Symptom Assessment Scale in children aged 7-12. *J Pain Symptom Manage.* 2002;23(1):10–16.

66. Wolfe J, Hammel JF, Edwards KE, et al. Easing of suffering in children with cancer at the end of life: is care changing? *J Clin Oncol.* 2008;26(10):1717–1723.

67. World Health Organization Website. *Cancer Control: Knowledge into Action: WHO Guide for Effective Programmes. Module 5-Palliative Care.* 2007. http://apps.who.int/iris/bitstream/10665/44024/1/9241547345_eng.pdf.

68. American Academy of Pediatrics. Committee on Bioethics and Committee on Hospital Care. Palliative care for children. *Pediatrics.* 2000;106(2):351–357.

69. Johnson LM, DeLario M, Baker J, Kane J. Palliative care in pediatrics. In: Berger A, Shuster Jr J, Von Roenn J, eds. *Palliative Care and Supportive Oncology.* 4th ed. Philadelphia, PA: Lippincott Williams & Wilkins; 2013:821–840.

70. Howlader N, Noone AM, Krapcho M, et al. *SEER Cancer Statistics Review, 1975-2013*National Cancer Institute Website; April 2016. http://seer.cancer.gov/csr/1975_2013/.

71. Smith TJ, Temin S, Alesi ER, et al. American Society of Clinical Oncology provisional clinical opinion: the integration of palliative care into standard oncology care. *J Clin Oncol.* 2012;30(8):880–887.

72. Lynn J, Adamson D. *Living Well at the End of Life: Adapting Health Care to Serious Chronic Illness in Old Age.* Santa Monica, CA: Rand; 2003.

73. Johnston DL, Nagel K, Friedman DL, et al. Availability and use of palliative care and end-of-life services for pediatric oncology patients. *J Clin Oncol.* 2008;26(28):4646–4650.

74. Roth M, Wang D, Kim M, Moody K. An assessment of the current state of palliative care education in pediatric hematology/oncology fellowship training. *Pediatr Blood Cancer.* 2009;53(4):647–651.

75. Wiener L, Zadeh S, Battles H, et al. Allowing adolescents and young adults to plan their end-of-life care. *Pediatrics.* November 2012;130(5):897–905.

76. National Institute for Mental Health. National Institute of Health Website. *Guide Offers Blueprint for End-of-Life Conversation with Youth.* December 28, 2012. https://www.nimh.nih.gov/news/science-news/2013/guide-offers-a-blueprint-for-end-of-life-conversation-with-youth.shtml.

77. Sommer D. Exploring the spirituality of children in the midst of illness and suffering. *Advocate.* 1994;1(2):7–12.

78. Hain RD, Miser A, Devins M, Wallace WH. Strong opioids in pediatric palliative medicine. *Paediatr Drugs.* 2005;7(1):1–9.

79. Friedrichsdorf SJ, Postier A, Dreyfus J, Osenga K, Sencer S, Wolfe J. Improved quality of life at end of life related to home-based palliative care in children with cancer. *J Support Oncol.* 2013;11(3):114–125.

80. Fraser LK, van Laar M, Miller M, et al. Does referral to specialist paediatric palliative care services reduce hospital admissions in oncology patients at the end of life? *Br J Cancer.* 2013;108(6):1273–1279.

81. Barfield R. Pediatric oncology and palliative care. *NC Med J.* 2014;75(4):276–277.

# CHAPTER 10

# Case Examples

MEAGAN B. FARMER, MS, CGC • NATHANIEL H. ROBIN, MD

## SCENARIOS

### Case 1

A 4-year-old female is being treated for adrenocortical carcinoma. Her pedigree is included below (Fig. 10.1).
- What is the differential based on the information provided?
- What, if any, testing would you begin with?
- If the most likely condition is confirmed, what management recommendations would you make for this patient and her family?

### Case 2

A 9-year-old boy presents with significant rectal bleeding and associated anemia. He is found to have six hamartomatous colorectal polyps on colonoscopy. His physical examination is negative. His pedigree is included below (Fig. 10.2).
- What is the differential based on the information provided?
- What, if any, further assessment and/or testing would you begin with?
- If the most likely condition is confirmed, what management recommendations would you make for this patient and his family?

### Case 3

A 6-week-old female presented with signs of impaired intestinal motility, including failure to pass meconium, constipation, and abdominal distention. Hirschsprung disease was confirmed with suction biopsies of the rectal mucosa and submucosa. A genetics consult was requested, and her physical examination was otherwise negative. Her parents were both present, and no dysmorphic features were noted. Her pedigree is below (Fig. 10.3).
- What are the potential etiologies to consider for Hirschsprung disease?[4]
- What should the work-up include?[4]
- If the most likely condition is confirmed, what management recommendations would you make for the patient and her family?

### Case 4

An 8-year-old male presents with pervasive developmental disorder not otherwise specified (autism).

His medical history is otherwise unremarkable. His pedigree is included below (Fig. 10.4). Chromosomal microarray and Fragile X testing were ordered by his pediatrician and were negative. Physical examination is only remarkable for macrocephaly (57 cm).
- What should the genetics work-up of autism include?
- Consider this case according to the proposed framework for evaluation.
- If the most likely condition is confirmed, what management recommendations would you make for the patient and his family?

## SOLUTIONS

### Case 1

A 4-year-old female is being treated for adrenocortical carcinoma. Her pedigree is included below (Fig. 10.1).
- What is the differential based on the information provided?
  - Li-Fraumeni syndrome (adrenocortical carcinoma, breast cancer)[1]
  - Beckwith-Wiedemann syndrome (adrenocortical carcinoma)[1]
  - BRCA-related hereditary breast and ovarian cancer (breast cancer)[2]
- What, if any, testing would you begin with?
  - Both adrenocortical carcinoma and early-onset breast cancer are associated with Li-Fraumeni syndrome.[1] Given this, TP53 sequencing and deletion/duplication analysis should be performed.
- If the most likely condition is confirmed, what management recommendations would you make for this patient and her family?
  - See Li-Fraumeni management recommendations in Chapter 6.
  - Neither parent has a personal history of cancer, but a TP53 mutation could have been inherited from either parent or be de novo. Parents should be offered testing, beginning with her father given the paternal grandmother's history of early-onset breast cancer.

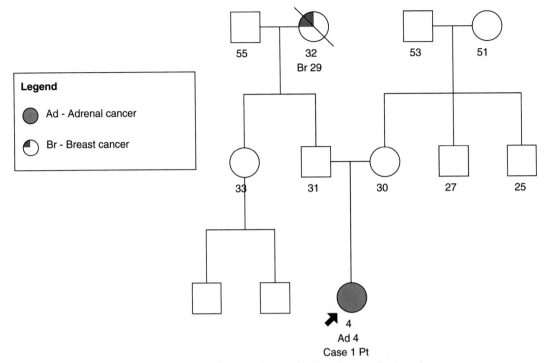

FIG. 10.1 A 4-year-old female being treated for adrenocortical carcinoma.

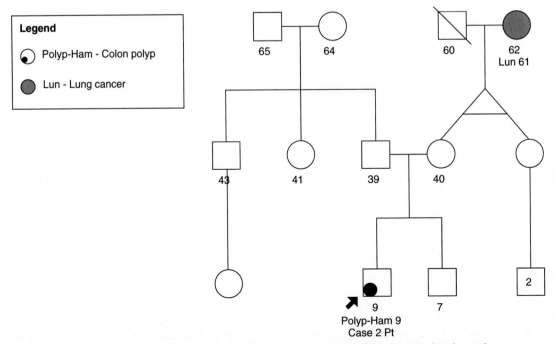

FIG. 10.2 A 9-year-old boy presents with significant rectal bleeding and associated anemia.

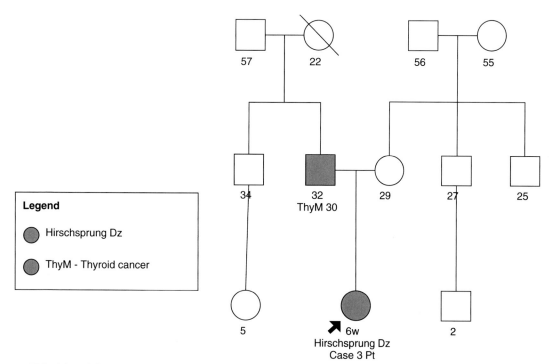

**Legend**

⬤ Hirschsprung Dz

⬤ ThyM - Thyroid cancer

FIG. 10.3 A 6-week-old female presented with signs of impaired intestinal motility, including failure to pass meconium, constipation, and abdominal distention.

## Case 2

A 9-year-old boy presents with significant rectal bleeding and associated anemia. He is found to have six hamartomatous colorectal polyps on colonoscopy. His physical examination is negative. His pedigree is included below (Fig. 10.2).
- What is the differential based on the information provided?
  - Juvenile polyposis syndrome (hamartomatous polyps with anemia)[3]
  - Cowden syndrome/PTEN hamartoma syndrome (hamartomatous polyps)[3]
  - Peutz-Jeghers syndrome (hamartomatous polyps)[3]
- What, if any, further assessment and/or testing would you begin with?
  - Review of colon polyp pathology to determine whether polyps appear to be juvenile type
    - If he has more than five juvenile-type polyps of the colorectum, he meets clinical diagnostic criteria for juvenile polyposis syndrome (see JPS section within Chapter 7 for more information).
  - Physical examination was reportedly negative. Confirm that head circumference is within normal limits and that there are no mucocutaneous findings suggestive of Peutz-Jeghers syndrome

to reduce suspicion for Cowden syndrome and Peutz-Jeghers syndrome, respectively.
- If the above assessment confirms suspicion of juvenile polyposis syndrome, perform BMPR1A and SMAD4 sequencing and deletion/duplication analysis. If a multigene panel, including analysis of several genes implicated in susceptibility to polyposis and/or colorectal cancer, is instead performed, note that you would likely be testing this patient for several conditions that are not associated with childhood onset.
- If the most likely condition is confirmed, what management recommendations would you make for this patient and his family?
  - See JPS management section within Chapter 6 for more information.
  - JPS can be due to inherited or de novo mutations. The patient's parents should be offered targeted testing.

## Case 3

A 6-week-old female presented with signs of impaired intestinal motility, including failure to pass meconium, constipation, and abdominal distention. Hirschsprung disease was confirmed with suction biopsies of the rectal mucosa and submucosa. A genetics consult was requested, and her physical examination was otherwise negative. Her parents were both present, and no dysmorphic features were noted. Her pedigree is below (Fig. 10.3).

- What are the potential etiologies to consider for Hirschsprung disease?[4]
  - Sporadic
  - Chromosomal causes (e.g., Down Syndrome)
  - Monogenic disorders
    - Nonsyndromic Hirschsprung disease
    - Syndromic Hirschsprung disease
- What should the work-up include?[4]
  - Detailed family history (Fig. 10.3)
    - Family history is remarkable for her father's history of medullary thyroid cancer, which raises suspicion for multiple endocrine neoplasia type 2 (MEN2).
  - Physical examination
    - Negative, reduces likelihood of many syndromic causes of Hirschsprung disease.
    - For more information, see GeneReviews Hirschsprung Disease Overview.[4]
  - Molecular genetic testing
    - Given her negative physical examination, family history of medullary thyroid cancer, and lack of signs of MEN2B in her parents

(see MEN2B section within Chapter 6 for more information), MEN2A or familial medullary thyroid cancer (FMTC) are most likely. RET testing should be performed. This can begin with sequencing of exons 10, 11, and 13–16 because most disease-causing mutations are located within these exons.[5] If this testing is negative, full sequence analysis could be performed reflexively. Alternatively, full RET sequencing could be considered as a first-line test.

- If the most likely condition is confirmed, what management recommendations would you make for the patient and her family?
  - See MEN2A/FMTC management section within Chapter 6 for more information.
  - The vast majority of cases of MEN2A/FMTC are due to a mutation that has been inherited from a parent.[5] Targeted testing should be offered to her father first, given this personal history of MTC.

## Case 4

An 8-year-old male presents with pervasive developmental disorder not otherwise specified (autism). His medical history is otherwise unremarkable. His pedigree is included below (Fig. 10.4).

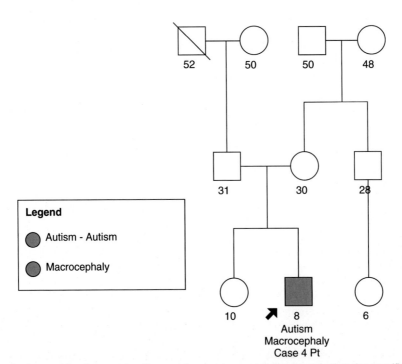

FIG. 10.4 An 8-year-old male presents with pervasive developmental disorder not otherwise specified (autism).

## REFERENCES

1. McKusick V, Tiller G. *OMIM Entry – # 202300-Adrenocortical Carcinoma, Hereditary; ADCC.* Omimorg; 2016. Available at: https://www.omim.org/entry/202300.
2. McKusick V, Hamosh A. *OMIM Entry – # 114480-Breast Cancer.* Omimorg; 2016. Available at: https://www.omim.org/entry/114480.
3. Haidle J, Howe J. *Juvenile Polyposis Syndrome.* Ncbinlmnihgov; 2016. Available at: https://www.ncbi.nlm.nih.gov/books/NBK1469/#jps.
4. Parisi M. *Hirschsprung Disease Overview.* Ncbinlmnihgov; 2016. Available at: https://www.ncbi.nlm.nih.gov/books/NBK1439/.
5. Marquard J, Eng C. *Multiple Endocrine Neoplasia Type 2.* Ncbinlmnihgov; 2016. Available at: https://www.ncbi.nlm.nih.gov/books/NBK1257/#men2.

## FURTHER READING

1. Schaefer G, Mendelsohn N. Clinical genetics evaluation in identifying the etiology of autism spectrum disorders: 2013 guideline revisions. *Genet Med.* 2013;15(5):399–407. http://dx.doi.org/10.1038/gim.2013.32.

# Index

*Note*: 'Page numbers followed by "f" indicate figures, "t" indicate tables and "b" indicate boxes.'

Printed in the United States
By Bookmasters